REASONABLE RATIONING

International Experience of Priority
Setting in Health Care

STATE OF HEALTH SERIES

Edited by Chris Ham, Professor of Health Policy and Management at the University of Birmingham and Director of the Strategy Unit at the Department of Health.

Current and forthcoming titles

REASONABLE RATIONING

International Experience of Priority
Setting in Health Care

EDITED BY
Chris Ham & Glenn Robert

Open University Press
Maidenhead · Philadelphia

Open University Press
McGraw-Hill Education
McGraw-Hill House
Shoppenhangers Road
Maidenhead
Berkshire
England
SL6 2QL

email: enquiries@openup.co.uk
world wide web: www.openup.co.uk

and
325 Chestnut Street
Philadelphia, PA 19106, USA

First Published 2003

A catalogue record of this book is available from the British Library

ISBN 0 335 21185 2 (pb)   0 335 21186 0 (hb)

Library of Congress Cataloging-in-Publication Data
Reasonable rationing: international experience of priority setting in health
care / edited by Chris Ham & Glenn Robert.
     p.   cm. – (State of health series)
  Includes bibliographical references and index.
  ISBN 0–335–21186–0 – ISBN 0–335–21185–2 (pbk.)
  1. Health care rationing – Developing countries. 2. Medical policy –
Developing countries. 3. Health planning – Developing countries. I. Ham,
Christopher. II. Robert, Glenn B., 1969– III. Series.
RA410.5. R425 2003
362.1′09712′4–dc21   2002035464

Typeset by RefineCatch Limited, Bungay, Suffolk
Printed in Great Britain by Bell and Bain Ltd, Glasgow

CONTENTS

SERIES EDITOR'S INTRODUCTION

Health services in many developed countries have come under critical scrutiny in recent years. In part this is because of increasing expenditure, much of it funded from public sources, and the pressure this has put on governments seeking to control public spending. Also important has been the perception that resources allocated to health services are not always deployed in an optimal fashion. Thus at a time when the scope for increasing expenditure is extremely limited, there is a need to search for ways of using existing budgets more efficiently. A further concern has been the desire to ensure access to health care of various groups on an equitable basis. In some countries this has been linked to a wish to enhance patient choice and to make service providers more responsive to patients as 'consumers'.

Underlying these specific concerns are a number of more fundamental developments which have a significant bearing on the performance of health services. Three are worth highlighting. First, there are demographic changes, including the ageing population and the decline in the proportion of the population of working age. These changes will both increase the demand for health care and at the same time limit the ability of health services to respond to this demand.

Second, advances in medical science will also give rise to new demands within the health services. These advances cover a range of possibilities, including innovations in surgery, drug therapy, screening and diagnosis. The pace of innovation quickened as the end of the twentieth century approached, with significant implications for the funding and provision of services.

Third, public expectations of health services are rising as those who use services demand higher standards of care. In part, this is stimulated by developments within the health service, including the availability of new technology. More fundamentally, it stems from the emergence of a more educated and informed population, in which people are accustomed to being treated as consumers rather than patients.

Against this background, policy makers in a number of countries are reviewing the future of health services. Those countries which have traditionally relied on a market in health care are making greater use of regulation and planning. Equally, those countries which have traditionally relied on regulation and planning are moving towards a more competitive approach. In no country is there complete satisfaction with existing methods of financing and delivery, and everywhere there is a search for new policy instruments.

The aim of this series is to contribute to debate about the future of health services through an analysis of major issues in health policy. These issues have been chosen because they are both of current interest and of enduring importance. The series is intended to be accessible to students and informed lay readers as well as to specialists working in this field. The aim is to go beyond a textbook approach to health policy analysis and to encourage authors to move debate about their issue forward. In this sense, each book presents a summary of current research and thinking, and an exploration of future policy directions.

Professor Chris Ham
Professor of Health Policy and Management at the University of Birmingham and Director, the Strategy Unit, Department of Health

LIST OF CONTRIBUTORS

Chris Ham is professor of health policy and management at the Health Services Management Centre, University of Birmingham. Since March 2000 he has been on secondment to the Department of Health, where he is director of the Strategy Unit. He was chair of the International Society on Priorities in Health Care from 1998 until 2000.

Glenn Robert is a senior research fellow at the Centre for Health Informatics and Multiprofessional Education, University College London. Prior to this he was a research fellow at the Health Services Management Centre, University of Birmingham.

Marc Berg is professor of social medical sciences at the Institute of Health Policy and Management at Erasmus University, Rotterdam.

Ashley Bloomfield has worked for the New Zealand National Health Committee (NHC) since 1997. He became NHC director in March 2000.

Angela Coulter is chief executive of the Picker Institute Europe. From 1993 until 1999 she was an executive director of the King's Fund in London, leading their work on health policy analysis, research and service development.

Douglas Martin is director of the Collaborative Programme in Bioethics, and assistant professor in the Department of Health Administration and the Joint Centre for Bioethics, University of Toronto. He is a member of the steering committee of the International Society on Priorities in Health Care.

Ole Frithjof Norheim is a general practitioner and associate professor in the section for Medical Ethics and the Philosophy of Science, Department of Public Health and Primary Health

Care and Centre for the Study of the Sciences and the Humanities at the University of Bergen.

Peter Singer is the Sun Life Financial Chair in Bioethics and director of the University of Toronto Joint Centre for Bioethics, and the programme director of the Canadian Program in Genomics and Global Health. He is also professor of medicine and practises internal medicine at Toronto Western Hospital.

Tom van der Grinten is professor of Health Care Policy and Organization at the Erasmus University Medical Center, Rotterdam.

1

INTRODUCTION
Chris Ham and Glenn Robert

This book is a contribution to the literature on health care rationing or priority setting, terms we use interchangeably throughout. The book extends work developed by one of us (CH) over the past decade. Initially this work focused on experience of priority setting in the UK National Health Service (NHS), drawing on the results of empirical research to describe and analyse how decision makers arrived at rationing decisions (Ham 1993). Subsequent contributions extended the analysis to encompass international experience of priority setting on the one hand (Ham 1995; Coulter and Ham 2000), and contested micro-level rationing decisions in the NHS on the other (Ham and Pickard 1998; Ham and McIver 2000). One of the points of similarity in these macro and micro studies was the attention given to the processes of decision making as well as the content of decisions.

As other writers have noted (for example, Klein *et al.* 1996), the interest in decision making processes arose from the difficulty of securing agreement on the principles that should guide decision making and the need therefore to ensure that the way in which decisions were reached was legitimate and fair. In this context, the argument of Daniels and Sabin (1998), that rationing decisions should demonstrate what they described as accountability for reasonableness, has received increasing attention. In essence, Daniels and Sabin argue that the need to set priorities is inevitable in both publicly and privately financed health care systems. This means that difficult choices have to be made, and in extreme cases access to services may be denied. Daniels and Sabin further argue that it is in the nature of priority setting decisions that there is likely to be disagreement among those involved. It follows that justice will only be served if there is due process in decision making.

On this basis, Daniels and Sabin outline the four conditions of accountability for reasonableness:

Publicity. Decisions must be publicly accessible.
Relevance. Rationales for decisions must rest on evidence that fair-minded parties agree are relevant.
Appeals. There is a mechanism for challenge and dispute resolution.
Enforcement. There is regulation of the process to ensure the first three conditions are met.

Early evidence suggested that accountability for reasonableness had relevance both in market-oriented systems such as the United States where it was developed and in publicly financed systems such as the United Kingdom (Ham 1999). What was less clear was the extent to which actual decision making met the conditions of accountability for reasonableness. To investigate this, we commissioned papers from authors in five countries to explore how decisions on health technologies were made in practice. These countries were chosen on pragmatic grounds, in particular the availability of experience and researchers relevant to the focus of this book. All of the countries have been at the forefront of efforts to set priorities more systematically, and the authors were invited to address the following seven questions in reporting their findings:

1. What procedures are used to determine whether health technologies should be funded?
2. What is the role of different institutions in these procedures?
3. What kind of evidence do these institutions expect/require/ consider in making funding decisions?
4. What standard of proof do they expect to be demonstrated in agreeing funding?
5. What appeal mechanisms are available for reviewing decisions?
6. What does experience in your country say about the debate between those who argue for stronger institutions and those who argue for better information to support priority setting?
7. To what extent does experience in your country meet the tests of accountability for reasonableness?

Using these questions as the starting point, the authors were invited to focus on the areas of greatest current interest in relation to priority setting in their own health care system.

The chapters in this book have gone through several drafts before publication. In this sense, the preparation of the book has involved a dialogue over a period of almost three years between the authors and the editors, and among the authors themselves. The core of the book comprises five chapters describing and analysing experience in each of the chosen countries. These country 'case studies' are preceded by an overview of international experience of rationing, and are followed by a concluding chapter that seeks to compare and contrast the evidence reported here and relate it back to Daniels and Sabin's framework. In this way, the book follows on from the papers presented at the Second International Conference on priority setting (Ham and Coulter 2000) and offers an up-to-date account of the state of the art of priority setting in a number of countries at the leading edge of work in this field.

Several debts have been incurred along the way. To begin with, we would like to thank GlaxoSmithKline for providing support in the form of an educational grant to enable the costs of writing the book to be covered. We are also grateful to Norman Daniels who read an earlier draft of the manuscript and supplied detailed comments and suggestions to the authors and editors. Thanks are due to the publishers of the *Journal of Health Services Research and Policy* for permission to publish an article by Chris Ham and Angela Coulter as Chapter 2 in this book, and to our colleagues at the Health Services Management Centre at the University of Birmingham who assisted in the organization of the research. Any errors or omissions remain the responsibility of the editors and authors.

2

INTERNATIONAL EXPERIENCE OF RATIONING[1]
Chris Ham and Angela Coulter

INTRODUCTION

In an era of ever-increasing medical possibilities, publicly financed health care systems face the challenge of determining what services should be covered for the insured population. This challenge, usually referred to as health care rationing or priority setting, words we shall use interchangeably, has led governments in a number of countries to take a more systematic approach to the determination of service coverage than has usually been the case in the past. Specifically, policy makers in these countries have encouraged explicit debate about priority setting, starting in the second half of the 1980s and continuing into the 1990s. In so doing, they have built on efforts to strengthen health technology assessment and to determine coverage of pharmaceuticals in order to address priority setting in the round.

One of the earliest examples was the state of Oregon, whose work to draw up a list of priorities for Medicaid as a way of expanding population coverage has been widely studied and reported (Strosberg *et al.* 1992). The experience of Oregon finds echoes in countries as diverse as Denmark, Finland, Norway, Sweden, the Netherlands, New Zealand, Israel and now the United Kingdom as policy makers seek to square the circle of increasing demands and limited resources (Coulter and Ham 2000). In all of these systems, work has been undertaken to develop more explicit approaches to rationing at a macro level in the recognition that diffusing blame and muddling through may no longer be sufficient. In parallel, there have been efforts to strengthen decision making at the meso and micro levels in the recognition that responsibility for rationing is located at many different points. This work can be seen as an attempt by policy makers to supplement political bargaining over the allocation of health care resources with efforts to puzzle more intelligently about priority setting. This chapter summarizes the results of these efforts and assesses the implications for those charged with making rationing decisions.

RATIONING ALL AROUND THE WORLD

Experience in states that have sought to be more systematic in their approach to determining what services should be covered for the insured population demonstrates the menu of possibilities available to health policy makers in setting priorities at a macro level. Despite the attention given in health policy debates to the development of a basic benefits package or a set of core services, only in Oregon's Medicaid programme has the priority setting dilemma been addressed mainly by excluding certain categories of treatments from funding. In Oregon this was done by drawing up a list of condition–treatment pairs and ranking these in order of priority.

When it was implemented in 1994, the Oregon Health Plan funded 565 out of 696 treatments, the main exclusions being treatments for minor medical conditions or those where evidence of effectiveness was lacking. In taking this approach, policy makers in Oregon were seeking to increase population coverage by limiting service coverage, although even the original Oregon Plan included some services that had previously been outside Medicaid, such as dental care. Subsequent revisions have tended to increase the scope of service coverage to the extent that most treatments are now covered (Bodenheimer 1997; Ham 1998; Jacobs *et al.* 1999). An example is cochlear implants, which were added to the list of funded services when new evidence on the benefits offered by implants became available.

Oregon aside, those responsible for rationing have adopted an approach centred on the development of national frameworks to guide priority setting rather than defined lists of treatments or services to be covered. The Netherlands and New Zealand exemplify this approach. In the Netherlands, politicians have shied away from the exclusion of services from funding, after flirting with this strategy. One of the reasons for their reluctance to go down the road of exclusions was criticism from groups opposed to the removal of services from funding. An example was the proposal to exclude funding of contraceptive pills from coverage, a proposal that was withdrawn after opposition from women's groups and family planning organizations. Similarly, in New Zealand the government-appointed Core Services Committee declined to draw up a list of services to be publicly funded, even though it was charged with this task. The view of the Committee was that priority setting was best approached not by limiting service coverage but by determining how services could be targeted on those patients most likely to benefit. In both the Netherlands and New Zealand, effort has focused on the development of evidence based guidelines intended to ensure that services are provided appropriately.

Research into explicit rationing at a macro level demonstrates that there are no simple or technical solutions that can resolve the dilemmas facing decision makers. As Oregon discovered, techniques drawn from economics designed to compare the costs and outcomes of health technologies are not sufficiently developed to provide a reliable basis for decision making (Hadhorn 1991). This was starkly illustrated by the ranking of tooth capping above appendectomy in the original Oregon list. Anomalous results of this kind show the difficulties of applying economic analysis in practice and also reveal gaps in the availability of information on costs and benefits.

Yet even if information were more complete, the results of economic analysis would still have to be interpreted by policy makers in the process of determining priorities, given that the aim of health policy is not simply to maximize health gain for the resources available. As an example, the pursuit of equity may result in resources being allocated to services where the cost of achieving a certain quantum of benefit is greater than in relation to alternatives. Trade-offs of this kind are made all the time in health policy and indicate the potential incompatibility of efficiency and equity objectives.

Those responsible for priority setting therefore have to confront the need to make decisions in conditions of incomplete information and likely conflicts between objectives. While one response has been to seek to fill the gaps in information and to refine the tools to support decision making, for example through an investment in health technology assessment and evidence based medicine, another approach has been to widen the debate beyond the experts (whether physicians or economists) to include other stakeholders. An important motivation in this context is that choices in health care involve making judgements about the relative priority to be attached to different objectives and services. It follows that these choices need to be informed by an understanding of community preferences, if they are to gain acceptance among those affected.

It was for this reason that decision makers in Oregon, for example, sought to strengthen their approach by drawing on public consultation and evidence of community values in determining priorities for Medicaid. Other systems have also endeavoured to engage the public in debate about rationing, and a wide range of methods have been used for this purpose. In part this has been stimulated by a concern to inform the public about the inevitability of rationing, and in part it has been designed to use the public's views to inform decision making.

The need to make trade-offs in health care rationing has also led to an interest in clarifying the values that should guide decision making. In some systems, such as the Netherlands, Oregon and Sweden, values have been defined explicitly, while in others they have emerged implicitly. The work done on values has been used to aid the process of rationing by identifying criteria for making choices and in some cases for ordering priorities. A distinctive feature of the Swedish approach is the attempt to rank values, the highest priority being attached to respect for human dignity followed by solidarity or equity and then by efficiency (Swedish Parliamentary Priorities Commission 1995). The experience of Sweden reinforces our earlier observation on the potential conflict between objectives.

With few exceptions, the articulation of values has remained a high-level activity, and little effort has been put into the use of values in decision making or in day-to-day clinical practice. As a consequence, there is often a gap between the proposals put forward by government committees and expert groups in relation to rationing and what happens at the meso and micro levels. This is most apparent in the case of countries such as Norway and Sweden where the emphasis has been placed on the promulgation of ethical frameworks at a macro level to guide decision making. The impact of such frameworks, based on the identification of core values rather than core services, is difficult to determine precisely because they are expressed in general terms and their effects have not been fully evaluated.

Set against this, explicit rationing may result in more resources being allocated to the health care budget if the approaches adopted are sufficiently specific to expose areas of underfunding and unmet need. This was one of the effects of the Oregon Health Plan, in that the legislature voted more resources for Medicaid to enable the cut-off point for funding to be lowered when the effects of maintaining previous funding levels became transparent. Similarly, in New Zealand the government provided extra funds to reduce waiting lists for surgery when it was possible to identify patients who would benefit from treatment but were not receiving it because of financial constraints. Experience in Israel reinforces this point, with the government there increasing the health care budget to enable new and relatively expensive drugs for cancer care to be included in the benefits package following publicity demonstrating the denial of treatment to patients (including children) in need (Chinitz *et al.* 1998).

THE POLITICS OF RATIONING

One clear conclusion from experience so far is the sheer messiness of health care decision making and the inherently political nature of priority setting. The allocation of scarce resources between competing demands is at once an economic challenge and a political puzzle. Giving higher priority to one service means giving low priority to another when budgets are fixed, and the evidence indicates that this is likely to stimulate lobbying among those groups affected. One of the reasons why political leaders have been reluctant to engage in explicit rationing at a macro level in the past is that in determining priorities they are also accepting responsibility for what may be unpopular choices. This helps to explain why politicians in most countries have declined to ration by excluding treatments or services from funding even though priority setting has become more explicit.

In these circumstances, there is a tendency for policy makers to seek to avoid blame either by ducking tough choices or by devolving responsibility to others. Rationing by guidelines rather than exclusions is one manifestation of this, in that it leaves ultimate responsibility for deciding who should be given access to health care resources to agencies such as sickness funds and health authorities at the meso level and to physicians at the micro level. The tendency of political leaders to avoid blame for rationing is consistent with research into the motivations of politicians (Weaver 1986). It is also congruent with the findings of research into comparative social policy demonstrating that retrenchment strategies are more likely to take the form of relatively incremental and invisible initiatives than direct cut-backs (Pierson 1994).

Partly because of this, but also because of the obstacles to developing more systematic approaches, some writers argue that muddling through is a virtue rather than a sin and, whatever its weaknesses, is to be preferred to the fruitless quest for a technical 'fix'. In other words, disillusion with the results of systematic attempts to set priorities is used to justify the *status quo ante* and to caution against the pursuit of more 'rational' solutions. This is the contention of, among others, Mechanic (1997), who argues that implicit decision making offers greater flexibility in circumstances in which judgements about treatments are surrounded by uncertainty and the needs of patients are diverse. Mechanic acknowledges that explicit approaches have a part to play at the macro and meso levels but, even so, he maintains that these approaches are liable to political manipulation and are not sufficiently responsive to change. Mechanic's view is endorsed by Hunter (1993), who contends that 'muddling through elegantly' is the most that can be expected and who is even more sceptical than Mechanic about the desirability of explicitness.

A related argument is advanced by Klein (1998), who is sympathetic to the case for muddling through but places greater emphasis on the need to strengthen the institutional basis of decision making. Writing as a policy analyst, Klein sees priority setting as 'inescapably a political process' in which debate and discussion between different interests are inevitable. It follows from this that the challenge is to devise mechanisms for addressing the intractable questions involved, while being cautious about the likelihood of finding answers. Klein is here echoing Holm's (1998) analysis of experience in the Nordic countries which points to the increasing interest in transparent and accountable decision making processes at a macro level rather than the pursuit of technical solutions.

As Holm (1998) shows, policy makers in these countries have turned their attention to ways of strengthening decision making processes to generate legitimacy for rationing as the limits of technical approaches have been exposed. Specifically, expert committees in both Denmark and Norway have made proposals for widening the debate about priority setting and involving a range of stakeholders. The importance of transparent and accountable decision making processes is reinforced by Daniels and Sabin's analysis of limit setting decisions in managed care organizations. On the basis of their analysis, Daniels and Sabin (1998) set out the four conditions presented in Chapter 1 that have to be met to demonstrate 'accountability for reasonableness'.

The relevance of these conditions has been demonstrated in studies of priority setting decisions in the United Kingdom as well as the United States, suggesting that the characteristics of defensible decision making apply regardless of differences in the funding and provision of health care. This was clearly illustrated by the case of Child B in which an English health authority that declined to fund further intensive treatment for a girl with end-stage leukaemia found itself vulnerable because of weaknesses in the decision making process (Ham and Pickard 1998). The common thread in both north American and European experience is the need to show that the way in which priorities are set is fair and reasonable even if agreement on the outcome is not possible. A similar motivation can be detected in New Zealand, where the work of the Core Services Committee (since renamed the National Health Committee) has given particular emphasis to raising public awareness of priority setting in health care and bringing choices out into the open (Edgar 2000). Having made this point, those involved in this work recognize that much remains to be done to promote public involvement in and understanding of priority setting. In other words, just as techniques drawn from economics and other disciplines are still in the process of development, so too methods of public participation and stakeholder debate need to be refined.

A NEW SYNTHESIS

To articulate these arguments is to illustrate that approaches to priority setting do not simply involve a choice between muddling through implicitly and pursuing systematic, explicit alternatives. Our reading of the international evidence is that these and related dichotomies fail to capture the complexity of rationing in practice. Put another way, the policy learning that has occurred in the decade or so since political leaders in Oregon and elsewhere grasped the nettle of explicit priority setting has highlighted not only the absence of technical solutions but also the need to join together approaches that have often been presented as alternatives (Martin and Singer 2000).

The argument can be taken a stage further by invoking the debate between Klein and Williams (2000) that formed the centrepiece of the Second International Conference on Priorities in Health Care. Writing as an economist, Williams challenged Klein's contention (see above) that strengthening the institutional basis of rationing was the issue that needed most urgent attention. Williams maintained that effective priority setting required clarity about objectives, information about costs and outcomes, and the ability to measure performance. In other words, Williams reasserted the case for technical solutions. For his part, Klein responded that the key task was less to refine the technical basis of decision making than to construct a process that enabled a proper discussion to occur given that questions of rationing 'cannot be resolved by an appeal to science'.

Our view is that the debate between Williams and Klein is a defining example of the false antitheses that have been so much in evidence in discussions in this field, even accepting that their respective positions may have been artificially polarized for the purpose of debate. The choice available to policy makers is not between more information and stronger institutions, rather it is a matter of how the work of institutions can be enhanced through the provision of better information and other mechanisms. Expressed in the language used earlier in this chapter, the challenge is to improve both technical approaches *and* decision making processes to enable the judgements that lie behind rationing to be as soundly based as possible. In relation to techniques, this means developing further the work of economists and others to inform decisions on priorities. And in relation to decision making processes, it entails developing institutions capable of using these techniques and also of involving the public and other stakeholders in debating priorities and making choices.

To make this point is to suggest that strengthening information and institutions also involves transcending another dichotomy, namely that concerning the role of experts and lay people in rationing. The challenge here is to find ways of enhancing the contribution of the public in its many different guises alongside that of experts. International experience testifies to the efforts that have been made to consult the public and to promote democratic deliberation in health care through the use of surveys, focus groups, consensus conferences and other methods. In parallel, the advice of experts has been drawn on through membership of government committees set up to advise on priority setting and use of the findings of evaluative research. A new synthesis requires that the input of both experts and lay people is seen as legitimate and relevant to decision making on priorities and that continuing efforts are made to find the most appropriate mechanisms for securing this input. This has recently been recognized in the United Kingdom with a proposal to set up a Citizens Council to advise the national agency charged with advising government on priority setting.

Similar considerations apply to the debate about the comparative advantages of explicit and implicit decision making. As experience shows, the choice between explicit and implicit rationing hinges on how political leaders deal with controversial choices when they arise. In the case of Israel, for example, an explicit approach to the determination of additions to the services that should be covered was combined with the imposition of limits on an implicit basis. Confirming our reading of international experience, analysts of this approach have concluded that 'The Israeli case suggests that explicit and implicit approaches to rationing and priority setting are not exclusive alternatives but rather complementary tools which support each other' (Chinitz *et al.* 1998).

Much the same applies in the United Kingdom, which is belatedly following the example of the other countries reviewed here through the establishment of the National Institute for Clinical Excellence (NICE) to advise politicians on priority setting. The modus operandi of NICE follows (unconsciously) the precepts of Daniels and Sabin, with a commitment to transparency and accountability in decision making on the funding of new technologies. This explicit approach goes hand in hand with a continuation of implicit decision making in many other aspects of rationing within the National Health Service (NHS), including the decisions that physicians make on the implementation of NICE guidelines and advice. Explicit rationing at a macro level is in this way combined with implicit rationing at a micro level. And at the meso level, health authorities have adopted both explicit and implicit approaches in discharging their responsibilities (Ham 1993; Klein *et al.* 1996; Hope *et al.* 1998).

The other element of the new synthesis is the use of exclusions as well as guidelines in addressing the priority setting dilemma. We have emphasized the political obstacles to rationing by exclusion, but in addition it has to be acknowledged that there are other reasons for avoiding this approach to priority setting. The weight of evidence suggests that there are few treatments that are wholly good or entirely bad, and the challenge for decision makers is to ensure that services are funded and provided to those patients who stand to benefit. This was expressed clearly by the chairman of the New Zealand Core Services Committee:

> The approach we decided to take was one that has flexibility to take account of an individual's circumstances when deciding if a service or treatment should be publicly funded. For example . . . instead of a decision that says hormone replacement therapy (HRT) is either core or non-core . . . the committee has decided

that in certain circumstances HRT will be a core service and in others it won't be. The committee has recommended that HRT be a core service where there is clinical and research-based agreement that it constitutes an appropriate and effective treatment.

(Jones 1993)

It is this that provides the rationale for the development of guidelines designed to target services and resources to achieve the most health gain for the population served. In reality, guidelines can be used alongside exclusions, as in the approach taken in the Netherlands which combines the exclusion of a limited number of services – examples being cosmetic surgery, adult dental care and homeopathic medicines – with the use of guidelines for the majority of services in a manner that is also finding favour elsewhere. Another example is the United Kingdom, where the exclusion of new drugs like Relenza from NHS funding is occurring at the margins, with the main emphasis being placed on the use of guidelines intended to ensure that those services that are funded are used appropriately and effectively. Indeed, in the United Kingdom, NICE has since reversed its original decision on Relenza and the drug can now be prescribed within defined guidelines. A further example is Oregon, where the inclusion of services on the list of funded treatments is accompanied by the use of guidelines to ensure that these services are provided appropriately. It might be added that setting priorities through guidelines preserves the degree of discretion in the treatment of individual patients that for Mechanic (1997) provides the basis for implicit rationing in health care.

Having made this point, it is important to recognize the force of Norheim's argument that guidelines themselves need to be developed through fair and open procedures. That is, the increasing reliance on guidelines in rationing requires the same rigour in relation to how guidelines are determined as decisions on whether or not to exclude services entirely from funding. Only in this way, Norheim argues, will it be possible to demonstrate that guidelines are acceptable and the decisions on which they are based defensible (Norheim 1999).

CONCLUSION

In conclusion, we return to address the other dichotomy that has run through this chapter, and that was identified by Heclo (1974) in a study of comparative social policy published over twenty years ago, namely the conception of policy making as a process of bargaining between interests on the one hand, and an exercise in puzzling and learning on the other. It is not necessary to subscribe to a view of policy making as red in tooth and claw to recognize the way in which debates about priority setting illustrate the quest for power and influence in the health sector. This is evident in the role of pressure groups in lobbying for additional resources for their priorities and the strategies used by political leaders to evade responsibility for unpopular choices. One of the conundrums in this context is the willingness of politicians to be brave (or foolish, depending on your point of view) in some systems, but not in others, by encouraging explicit rationing at the macro level. The point here, to reiterate our earlier argument, is that explicitness tends to enhance accountability by making transparent the location of decisions and runs counter to the blame avoidance strategies that often motivate politicians.

Having made this point, there is evidence of learning in the policy process, exemplified by the retreat from purely technical solutions and the efforts made to involve the public in debates on rationing. There is also an increasing focus, in what Holm (1998) describes as the second phase of priority setting, on the process of determining priorities. The interest in decision making processes is at once a response to the shortcomings of technical solutions and an attempt to earn legitimacy for what will often be difficult choices. Furthermore, by widening the circle of participants in decision making and demonstrating that the way in which decisions are made is rigorous and fair, those responsible for rationing are, consciously or unconsciously, striving to achieve accountability for reasonableness in the rationing process.

There is also evidence of learning in the partial retreat from explicitness in some countries. The renewed (in some cases, continuing) focus on the meso and micro levels of rationing can be interpreted as a return to blame avoidance as decision makers respond to the costs of being explicit about priorities at the macro level by shifting the emphasis and responsibility to agencies such as sickness funds and health authorities and to physicians. If this interpretation is correct, then the recent interest in explicit rationing may be a temporary aberration in a much longer history of muddling through and evading responsibility. In other words, the political costs of explicitness may outweigh the benefits, and this could result in a return to previous decision making processes.

The force of this observation is underlined by experience in those countries like the United States that (with limited exceptions such as Oregon) have chosen not to ration explicitly. As the US experience suggests, there remain fundamental political obstacles to adopting a different approach, not least because 'the American way of rationing is to decentralize (in political terms hide) the choices; the result is rationing through an accumulation of narrow public policies, private decisions and luck' (Morone 1992). This is because in the US 'attempts to ration health care explicitly are political dynamite' (Morone 1992). Nevertheless, decisions about limits to coverage and whether to fund new technologies have to be taken. In the US these decisions fall to public agencies, insurers and managed care organizations. Whether they like it or not, these agencies are involved in rationing (Daniels 2000; Rodwin 2000).

In both the US and elsewhere, the release of the rationing genie from the bottle has had the effect of initiating a debate that will be difficult to halt. At a time when there is increasing public awareness of the possibilities created by medical advances and the denial of access to treatment, the challenge is not how to avoid discussion of rationing at the macro level, but rather how to develop an informed democratic consensus model in which through broad mechanisms of public deliberation there is debate about how limited health care resources can be distributed. The rationale for encouraging democratic deliberation is that choices in health care involve moral issues that should be neither hidden nor fudged (Fleck 1992). If those responsible for rationing continue to obfuscate and fail to confront the dilemmas directly, then public confidence in the legitimacy of decisions and those charged with making them will be further undermined. In this sense, the case for a systematic approach is at root an argument to maintain and in some cases restore faith in the political system and to strengthen democratic practices. It is also an argument for finding a way of increasing the resources available for health care in the light of evidence that explicitness makes it more difficult for policy makers to evade responsibility for difficult choices.

NOTE

1 This chapter originally appeared as: Ham C and Coulter A (2001). Explicit and implicit rationing: taking responsibility and avoiding blame for health care choices. Journal of Health Services Research and Policy, 6(3): 163–9.

3

NEW ZEALAND
Ashley Bloomfield[1]

INTRODUCTION

Making decisions about who does – or does not – receive health care services has been a feature of health care systems for decades. More recently, these decisions have been the subject of international interest as all developed countries have grappled with rising health care costs and the need to ration health services explicitly. One central aspect of priority setting is the evaluation of new health technologies, defined very broadly as any new intervention (including a new use for an existing technology), procedure or programme. The purpose of this chapter is to describe the institutions involved in decisions about new technologies in New Zealand and the processes they employ to assess new technologies.

In order to set the scene, the major milestones in the development of priority setting processes are first outlined. Drawing on this description, as well as the specific consideration of new technology assessment, the discussion focuses on two issues:

- What does New Zealand experience say about the debate between those who argue for stronger institutions and those who argue for better information to support priority setting (and other decision making)?
- To what extent does the current New Zealand situation fulfil Daniels and Sabin's (1998) four conditions of 'accountability for reasonableness'?

As the author's experience is largely at the macro level, the processes and institutions described are predominantly at this level.

A BRIEF OVERVIEW OF THE NEW ZEALAND
HEALTH SYSTEM

The New Zealand health system encompasses both health and disability support services and is largely publicly funded through general taxation. New Zealand's total health expenditure as a proportion of gross domestic product was 8.5 per cent in 1999/2000. The proportion of health expenditure from public funding declined in the early 1990s but has stabilized at approximately 78 per cent of total health expenditure (Table 3.1) (Ministry of Health 2002). About 34 per cent of the population have private health insurance, a decline from 51 per cent in 1990 (Health Funds Association of New Zealand 1999). This insurance is largely to cover elective surgery and primary care co-payments, and accounts for only 6.3 per cent of total health expenditure. Private household expenditure accounted for 15.4 per cent of total health expenditure in 1999/2000.

Table 3.1 Total health funding in 1979/80 and 1999/2000 (per cent)

Year	1979/80	1999/2000
Publicly funded	88.1	78.5
Privately funded	11.9	22.0

Source: Ministry of Health (2002).

Care in public hospitals is free, while subsidies for primary care (largely general practice) are means-tested. As only 60 per cent of general practitioners' income is sourced from public funding, there are significant co-payments for primary care for most people. Care for injuries is publicly funded through a 'no-fault' national accident compensation scheme, which differs from other health care in that it is entitlement-based; there are also co-payments for treatment of injuries in primary care.

The health sector was restructured following the election of a centre-left Labour–Alliance coalition government in November 1999. Figure 3.1 identifies, and shows the relationships between, the main health sector organizations in New Zealand. Public hospitals are run by 21 district health boards (DHBs), which also have responsibility for purchasing many health services in their regions. General practices in New Zealand are largely privately owned, although not-for-profit 'third sector' providers provide an increasing proportion of primary care.

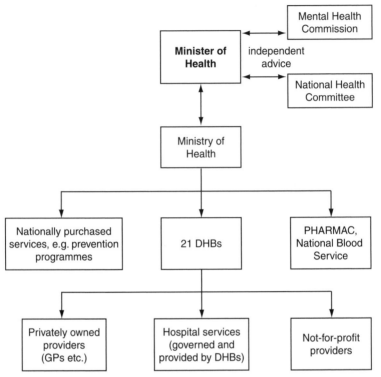

Figure 3.1   The publicly funded health and disability support system in New Zealand

Before 2001, the main difference was a purchaser–provider split with a separate national funder, the Health Funding Authority (HFA). The latter was established through the amalgamation of four regional health authorities in 1998. The passing of new legislation in December 2000 saw the dissolution of the HFA, with its functions split between an enlarged Ministry of Health and the 21 DHBs. The latter are now responsible for purchasing and providing services for their geographical populations in order to achieve health goals outlined in a 'New Zealand Health Strategy' (Minister of Health 2000). In addition, they provide hospital-based services in their regions. The national funding role passed to the Ministry of Health, with a staged devolution to the DHBs which commenced in July 2001.

Life expectancy at birth has improved during the past four decades in New Zealand. In 1997, women lived to an average age of 79.6

years, and men lived to an average age of 74.3 years. The main causes
of death are cardiovascular disease and cancer. Over the past two
decades, life expectancy for Maori (the indigenous people of New
Zealand) has increased significantly, and Maori infant mortality
rates have continued to decline. However, Maori life expectancy and
mortality rates are still worse than those of non-Maori. Maori tend
to have higher death rates than non-Maori in most disease areas,
including diabetes, lung cancer and cardiovascular disease; for
example, the mortality from diabetes for Maori is almost six times
that of non-Maori.

A BRIEF HISTORY OF PRIORITY SETTING IN
NEW ZEALAND

Priority setting in New Zealand arrived on the health policy agenda
in the early 1990s. Wide-ranging reforms at that time established an
'internal market', creating both a funder–provider split for the entire
sector and a funder–owner split for public hospitals. The reforms
also established a Core Services Committee, now the National
Health Committee (NHC).[2] As the original name suggests, the Committee was charged with advising the Minister of Health on the types
of 'care' that should be publicly funded and their relative priorities,
having due regard for available resources. A key task of the Committee was to advance public debate and understanding of limited
health care resources and the need to make choices about which
services would be funded and for whom.[3]

The National Health Committee's work: major milestones

Major milestones in the NHC's work over the past eight years have
been:

- the rejection of an Oregon-style list and agreement on prioritization principles;
- the development of booking systems to replace waiting lists; and
- the promulgation of guidelines and clinical priority access criteria.

Rejection of an Oregon-style list

In its third report to government in 1994, the Committee rejected the
use of a simple list to define the services to which New Zealanders

should have free access (National Advisory Committee on Core Health and Disability Support Services 1994). The Committee concluded that, rather than narrowly define which services should be publicly funded, there should be discussion about whether and when particular services should be offered. To assist this debate, the Committee proposed four priority setting principles that have underpinned much of its subsequent work (National Health Committee 1997):

• The treatment or service provides benefit (effectiveness).
• The treatment or service is value for money (efficiency).
• The treatment or service is a fair use of public funding (equity).
• The treatment or service is consistent with communities' values (acceptability).

While these high-level principles have informed the Committee's work, the NHC is only an advisory body. At issue is whether the processes in which these principles (or others) are applied are transparent so that we can see what they mean in the context of actual decisions (Daniels, personal communication). Subsequent discussion will address this issue.

Booking systems

The Committee's initial health-sector 'stocktake' identified widespread regional variations in access to elective procedures. In its second report, the Committee advocated the replacement of waiting lists for non-urgent procedures with booking systems. Under the latter, patients should have similar access to elective services, regardless of where they live, and be given a definite date for specialist services. There is a maximum time of six months for first specialist assessment, and surgery must be carried out within six months of decision to treat.

Booking systems have been implemented, although over a much longer period of time than initially envisaged and not without resistance from some secondary care providers and professionals (Hefford and Holmes 1999). Key elements of the booking systems are nationally consistent referral guidelines and clinical priority assessment criteria (discussed below). The former are developed by primary and secondary care physicians and include information about appropriate management of common conditions, guidance about when to refer and what information to provide. Currently, most of these guidelines are developed through a consensus process, with the intention of moving to a more explicitly evidence based process over time.

Guidelines and clinical priority access criteria

The Committee also provided leadership to the sector on the development and implementation of practice guidelines. Early Committee work on practice guidelines entailed the development of 17 guidelines through consensus conferences. In 1996, the Committee established a programme to train professionals and consumers to develop and implement more rigorous evidence based guidelines (also known as clinical practice or best practice guidelines). A number of national practice guidelines were also developed and disseminated to professionals under this programme.

The implementation of booking systems for elective services led to a stream of work on clinical priority access criteria (CPAC) in conjunction with the four regional health authorities (funders). CPAC are developed by specialist physicians and consist of an agreed collection of signs, symptoms and investigations that are considered to predict accurately and consistently the likely benefit an individual will receive from a particular procedure. The development of CPAC for coronary artery bypass grafting in New Zealand has been fully described (Hadhorn and Holmes 1997a, 1997b).

Other key prioritization developments

Following the 1993 New Zealand health reforms, the purchasing function was split between four regional health authorities which were merged into a single national Health Funding Authority (HFA) in late 1998. The HFA was responsible for purchasing the full range of personal health, public health and disability support services for New Zealanders. The Pharmaceutical Management Agency (PHARMAC), a Crown entity directly accountable to the Minister of Health, funds pharmaceutical products. Both the HFA and PHARMAC developed processes to assist in defining exactly what services and drugs should be publicly funded.

The Health Funding Authority prioritization process

Given the need to ensure that the best mix of services is purchased, much of the work of the HFA was predicated on prioritization. The move to a single funder provided considerable impetus for improving the processes for deciding what services should be purchased.

The process of deciding the best mix of services is complex and contains a number of inherent tensions and constraints. In the first instance, the government 'ring-fences' budgets for broad service areas, which can have direct operational implications around prioritization. This is a mechanism for helping to implement government policy on priority service areas, the principal goal being to protect funding for some areas, such as mental health and public health, to prevent their diversion to the funding of personal health services, where most of the cost pressure is. There are also ministerial policy directives about services that the HFA was required to fund, sometimes without additional tagged funding.

The HFA was required to consult with communities over their priorities, which must be balanced against the stated priorities of the government. While remaining responsive to local concerns and priorities, the HFA had to consider national consistency and strive to minimize inequities in access to services between groups or regions. Following its establishment, the HFA developed a more systematic and explicit process of prioritization. The HFA consulted widely with organizations and professionals in mid-1998 and proposed a prioritization process that combined a principle-based approach with the marginal analysis phase of programme budgeting and marginal analysis (PBMA) (Health Funding Authority 1998). The principles advocated by the HFA were efficacy, cost, equity (of outcome), acceptability and Maori health. With the exception of the addition of Maori health, these principles are identical to those espoused by the NHC since 1993.

The 'Maori health' principle stems from the government's obligation, imparted by the Treaty of Waitangi, to maintain and improve Maori health. The 1840 Treaty is widely regarded as New Zealand's founding document and establishes the basis for the relationship between the Maori and the Crown. The principles of the Treaty – partnership, participation and protection – have been articulated since the mid-1980s as central to decision making in the publicly funded health sector.

There is accumulating evidence of persistent relative inequalities in both access to health services and health status between Maori and non-Maori. This has focused efforts from the highest levels of government downward, and the HFA's inclusion of a specific Maori health principle reflected this. There is also clear acknowledgement of the need to address wider social and economic determinants in order to reduce health inequalities. The Maori health principle was to be incorporated and addressed at all levels of the analysis during the prioritization process, as well as facilitating opportunities for Maori to be involved in the design and provision of services or technologies being analysed (Health Funding Authority 1998).

During 1999/2000, the HFA 'prioritization process' was applied across the organization in bidding for the increase in funding available for 2000/01.[4] Both demand-driven proposals (e.g. expected increases in pharmaceutical and General Medical Subsidy spending) and new initiative proposals were subjected to the same process. A clear process was developed that required information relating to each of the five principles to be provided for technical and managerial review by groups drawn from across the organization. The only external review was from the Ministry of Health and Office of the Minister of Health, the purpose being to ensure consistency with government priorities and objectives.

The main weakness of the HFA's prioritization process was that the principles were not publicly consulted on. Its further usefulness, particularly within the new health system structure, will depend on its wide acceptance, and this will be difficult to achieve without adequate public consultation. The mechanism to do this now exists through the DHBs which are intended to be close to their communities and involve them in identifying priorities and making decisions. A further issue was that application of the process was resource-intensive in terms of the time involved in assessing the new proposals.

There were several other initiatives within the HFA that improved the prioritization of funding for services. These include separate 'high-cost treatment' and 'exceptional circumstances' budgets, which have their own access criteria. Over the past few years, purchase frameworks for hospital services have been developed that are generating agreement about reasonable and sustainable costs and volumes. This has greatly improved the information that is necessary to redirect funds towards priorities and to address regional inequities.

PHARMAC

The role of PHARMAC is to manage the national Pharmaceutical Schedule. The Schedule is a list, updated monthly, of over 3000 subsidized prescription drugs and related products. The PHARMAC board makes the final decision on subsidy levels and prescribing guidelines and conditions, with contributions from independent and medical experts on a Pharmacology and Therapeutics Advisory Committee and its specialist sub-committees, and PHARMAC's managers and analysts (PHARMAC 1999a). This process is outlined in more detail below.

PHARMAC has been highly successful in controlling increases in public expenditure on pharmaceuticals. While most developed countries continue to experience significant real growth in pharmaceutical expenditure, New Zealand's total publicly funded expenditure actually declined by 8 per cent between 1997 and 1998, and is still below the 1998 level (PHARMAC 2001).

Where is New Zealand's public debate on prioritization?

New Zealand has been a party to the international debate about rationing and priority setting in health care since the early 1990s. New Zealand has been included in previous inter-country comparisons of general priority setting processes (Honigsbaum *et al.* 1995, 1997), and New Zealanders have participated actively in the first three international conferences on priority setting (Feek *et al.* 1999; Edgar 2000; Oortwijn and Mulder 2000). As a result, New Zealand is considered by some international commentators to be one of the 'leading bunch' in the move to explicit priority setting. Certainly, progress has been made and many clinicians are now more conscious of the trade-offs that need to be made in deciding which people should or should not receive services. There is some evidence that public understanding has also matured somewhat, although this is much harder to gauge.

Two high-profile cases in 1995 and 1997, both about access to renal dialysis in end-stage renal failure, have been the focus for public and media discussion about rationing. These cases have been well documented, as have the range of opinions expressed by mainstream newspapers at the time (Feek *et al.* 1999). In the first case, the initial decision to deny dialysis on clinical grounds was rescinded after 'clinical review', in the face of widespread media attention. Two years later, and after the development of clinical guidelines for access to dialysis that had national clinical agreement, a similar decision (on clinical grounds) was upheld after several legal challenges, again in the face of close media scrutiny and active participation in the debate by some Members of Parliament.

HOW ARE DECISIONS ABOUT NEW HEALTH TECHNOLOGIES MADE PRESENTLY?

As for all prioritization decisions, those about new technologies are made at all levels of the New Zealand health system. Three 'generic' levels are considered – policy advice, purchasing/funding, and service provision – to outline how assessment of new technologies occurs. The processes that are used by the main institutions involved in making such decisions are outlined, and a summary of the kind of evidence required by each institution and appeals mechanisms for reviewing decisions are also described.

Policy advice and new technology assessment: the Ministry of Health and National Health Committee

The Ministry is the principal provider of health policy advice to the government. The introduction of some new technologies is subject to a formal policy appraisal process. For example, this has applied in recent years to the introduction of new vaccines, such as acellular pertussis vaccine (Box 3.1; see also Mansoor and Reid 1999), and screening programmes such as those for breast cancer (Members of the Breast Screening Policy Advisory Group 1998) and hepatitis B (Blakely and Thornley 1999).

Generally, the assessment of new technologies by the Ministry of Health at a policy level follows a lengthy process that includes the systematic evaluation of efficacy and cost-effectiveness evidence (Box 3.2). The highest grade of evidence available is sought, including systematic reviews or meta-analyses and cost-effectiveness

---

Box 3.1   Acellular pertussis vaccine

In the case of acellular pertussis vaccine a multidisciplinary standing committee, the Immunisation Advisory Committee (IAC), assessed the evidence and made recommendations to the Ministry regarding the introduction of the vaccine. The recommendations were accepted and the vaccine has become part of the free child immunization schedule. The deliberations of groups such as the IAC are not divorced from the decision making processes of the Ministry; officials actively participate in the meetings and work between meetings to collate further information and integrate the work of the groups into the policy development process.

Box 3.2   Breast screening

As in many other countries, population-based breast screening was introduced in New Zealand during the 1990s. Given the intensely political nature of breast screening, the process of assessing and introducing this 'new technology' was relatively transparent and systematic. A working group originally assessed the evidence in 1987 and recommended that a decision about routine screening be delayed until pilot programmes were established, with assessment of their effectiveness, economic efficiency and social acceptability (Skegg *et al.* 1988). Two pilot programmes commenced in the early 1990s. The performance of the pilot programmes was closely monitored, and they were formally evaluated after each two-year screening round. Information from the evaluation informed subsequent policy development and costing estimates for a national programme. Based on results of the pilots a nationwide free screening programme was announced by the Minister of Health in May 1995. A multi-disciplinary advisory group met between July 1995 and June 1996 to provide policy advice on the establishment of the national programme which was implemented between 1997 and 1999 for women aged 50–64 years. As expected, there has been pressure from various groups (notably professionals) to extend the age range for eligibility for free screening. Currently, efforts have focused on implementing the programme as effectively as possible to ensure the expected benefits are realized.

---

studies where available. Frequently, an 'expert' reference group is asked to assess this evidence and other relevant information and recommend appropriate action. The 'expertise' of Maori, Pacific Islands and consumer representatives on such groups is now widely accepted as essential.

The Ministry has only recently adopted a principle-based approach to decision making about priorities or the assessment of new health technology. This is in contrast to the HFA, whose process the Ministry inherited, and the NHC (discussed below). However, the Ministry does consider efficacy and cost-effectiveness evidence, and equity and acceptability issues are invariably examined. In addition, the Ministry usually consults widely with sector organizations, Maori, relevant communities and other central government agencies in formulating its advice.

As the prime agent of the Minister of Health, the Ministry must respond to the wishes of the Minister and Parliament. Thus, even the most rigorous evidence-informed policy analysis might be ignored for political reasons by the government, which might decide to fund a new technology despite contrary advice from the Ministry. The introduction of hepatitis B screening in New Zealand exemplifies this. In this instance, a decision was made by the government to fund a national hepatitis B screening programme despite well-advanced planning for a pilot programme and opposition to a national programme from the Ministry of Health, the HFA and the Treasury (Blakely and Thornley 1999). Official documents reveal that this policy reversal was the result of intense lobbying by an advocacy group, the Hepatitis Foundation, of Members of Parliament belonging to a minor coalition partner in the government of the day. Given that New Zealand is a democracy not a technocracy, such 'political interference' can be viewed as quite appropriate – the democratic process at work, where even the most rigorous, evidence-informed policy analysis is informed by the community's values expressed through the political process.

The processes used by the Ministry to make decisions about new technologies, such as screening programmes, are open to input by all stakeholders. Parties that disagree with decisions usually actively lobby the Minister of Health and other Members of Parliament and use the media to register their displeasure. The hepatitis B screening example demonstrates that sometimes this is successful. Of course, as such decisions become the policy of the government of the day, the issues are often raised during pre-election campaigning.

The National Health Committee, previously discussed, provides a second stream of policy advice. A portion of the Committee's advice relates to new technologies. The NHC provides independent advice to the Minister of Health who then seeks comment from other agencies – predominantly the Ministry of Health – before acting on the Committee's advice. Similarly to the Ministry of Health, the NHC's advice on new health technologies usually relates to matters such as screening programmes – for example, population screening for prostate cancer with prostate-specific antigen (PSA) and colorectal cancer with faecal occult bloods (see Box 3.3).

Before recommending that a new technology be funded, the Committee assesses the technology against four criteria: effectiveness, equity, acceptability and efficiency. A number of methods are used to develop Committee advice, but common to all is the systematic assessment of available evidence, as befits an organization that has championed evidence based practice. Thus, a high 'standard of proof' is required.

Box 3.3   Screening for prostate and colorectal cancer

In 1996, the NHC established a multidisciplinary working party to assess the potential risks and benefits of population screening for prostate cancer based on international evidence. The working party concluded that there was, at the time, no evidence to show that routinely screening men for prostate cancer prevents premature death from the disease, or that early detection and treatment of prostate cancer results in improved quality of life for men who have prostate cancer. Based on the work of this group, the Committee advised the Minister of Health that 'screening for prostate cancer in pre-symptomatic men is not an effective use of public health funds' (National Health Committee 1996).

The Committee was simultaneously represented on the Australian Health Technology Advisory Committee (AHTAC), which offered the same advice and had it accepted by the Australian Minister of Health. This culminated in a joint policy statement, advising against routine prostate screening for men without symptoms, being issued publicly by the NHC in New Zealand and the Minister for Health and Human Services in Australia on 12 August 1996. This advice was also consistent with that offered to governments in Canada, Europe and the USA.

A similar process was followed in 1998 to formulate advice on population screening for colorectal cancer. An expert working party was set up to review scientific evidence on the benefits, risks and adverse effects of a variety of screening methods. Large randomized controlled trials in the UK and Denmark had shown that screening with faecal occult blood tests could reduce colorectal cancer deaths. However, the working party recommended that population-based screening should not be introduced to New Zealand at that time, given the modest potential benefit, the considerable commitment of health resources required, and the fact that (follow-up) colonoscopy carries a small but real risk of harm. The working party's advice was endorsed by the NHC and passed to the Minister of Health. As with other Committee advice, a full report was also published (National Health Committee 1998). Further work has defined high-risk groups that the working party felt would benefit from screening, and that should have access to publicly funded surveillance and management.

In recent years, the Committee has provided advice to the Minister on screening for prostate cancer and colorectal cancer. The decision making processes for advice to the Minister on these issues differed from those conducted by the Ministry on breast cancer and hepatitis

B screening. In particular, the government may reject the Committee's advice but, as an independent advisory committee, the NHC is not subject to political interference while developing its advice.

As the Committee's work is tendered as 'free and frank' advice to the Minister, the Committee itself has no appeals process to review its decisions. Given the Committee's legislative requirement to consult, a wide range of feedback is sought and received when developing its advice. Organizations, newspaper editors and individuals who disagree with the Committee's advice do not hesitate to voice their concerns; the advice to reject population screening for prostate cancer continues to generate ministerial correspondence and periodic criticism in the media five years later.

New technology assessment by service purchasers and funders

Ministry of Health and District Health Boards (previously Health Funding Authority)

The HFA's prioritization process (described earlier) is still the framework for deciding which new services will be purchased. In the future, DHBs will be the main locus of decisions around funding for new (non-pharmaceutical) technologies. DHBs have already received information and instructions on applying the prioritization framework, and several have done so as part of annual planning for 2002/03. When developed and applied by the HFA, the prioritization process included new initiatives. However, the list of those projects that received a high priority for funding in recent years shows that few of them were actually new technologies (Health Funding Authority 1999a).

During the application of the prioritization process by the HFA during 1999/2000, two 'demonstration' projects were undertaken to help refine and test the prioritization framework and associated methodologies. These involved in-depth application of the framework, and one of them was a new technology assessment – a cost–utility analysis of deep brain stimulation as a new surgical intervention for Parkinson's disease (see Box 3.4; see also Health Funding Authority 1999b). The latter example demonstrates the application of a systematic, principle-based approach to assessing new technologies resulting in the conclusion that the new technology should not be funded. Yet, while the funding application was rejected on an ongoing basis, one procedure was approved as a one-off high-cost exceptional circumstance purchase (Health Funding Authority

---

Box 3.4   Evaluation of deep brain stimulation (DBS)

This involved a full cost–utility analysis, performed as part of the wider process for evaluating new technologies. At the time, the HFA purchased the alternative surgical intervention (unilateral pallidotomy) but a hospital applied for funding to perform DBS on the basis that it was a superior intervention.

The analysis indicated that unilateral pallidotomy is approximately 4.5 times more cost-effective than DBS, and sensitivity analysis did not alter the findings. Thus, the funding application was rejected. There was no additional consideration of the HFA's equity, acceptability or Maori health principles as it was felt to be unlikely that this would change the decision.

1999b), with suitable media adulation. This demonstrates that systematic, principle-based technical evaluation was not the only input into funding decisions by the HFA, even in the presence of an apparently 'clear-cut' result as this.

In general, the evaluation of new health technologies by the HFA did not follow a single uniform process. There was often little choice on the part of the HFA as to whether it chose to fund new technologies. Such decisions may be taken at a political or policy level, as in the case of the breast screening programme and the introduction of acellular pertussis vaccine, respectively. However, in these cases, the HFA was part of the decision making process and usually specific additional funding was tagged for new or additional services.

Aside from the efforts of individual advisers, there is no formal 'horizon scanning' activity, that is, deliberate and proactive scanning for potential new technologies or new uses for existing technologies. New technology evaluation is often prompted by approaches from health care providers or consumer groups. Until recently, the process for considering these requests was *ad hoc*, although this is not to say that a high standard of proof was not required. As this has become the principal route for considering whether or not to (explicitly) fund new technologies, the HFA developed a more formal application and prioritization process for new technologies. The application process has been adapted from that used by the Australian Medicare Services Advisory Committee (see Box 3.5) and decisions are predicated on the HFA's five decision making principles, previously discussed.

New Zealand does have a health technology assessment capacity, New Zealand Health Technology Assessment (NZHTA), which is

---

Box 3.5   HFA new technologies/services application

The application form consists of 13 sections:

1. Applicant details
2. Description of the new technology and compliance with any regulatory requirements
3. Commercial-in-confidence material
4. Indication for use of the new technology
5. Public health significance and patient selection
6. Where the new technology will be used and by whom
7. Comparable existing service
8. Estimated utilization
9. Summary of literature
10. Evaluation of evidence
11. Economic evaluation
12. Additional clinical opinion
13. Endorsement from medical college/specialist society or other professional organization.

---

part of the International Network of Agencies for Health Technology Assessment (INAHTA). Established in 1997, NZHTA is funded by the Ministry of Health and its work programme is largely determined by the Ministry's needs. However, until recently there was no systematic process to assess and prioritize requests for reviews by the NZHTA. This has resulted in the NZHTA being asked sometimes to answer ill-defined questions, many of which are focused on service configuration rather than the effectiveness or cost-effectiveness of specific interventions or programmes.

Many staff at the Ministry (and HFA previously) have a limited knowledge of the value that the NZHTA function can add to its work, in particular a more systematic approach to assessing new health technologies. The example on nuchal translucency screening in Box 3.6 illustrates a lost 'opportunity' in this regard.

In summary, while there is still no uniform process for funding decisions for new technologies, Ministry and DHB (and previously HFA) funding decisions around new technologies usually require a high level of evidence: randomized controlled trial evidence for efficacy where possible, and at least some cost–benefit information. A more formal process has been introduced recently that has improved the standard of proof required. Thus, while funding and prioritization decisions continue to be influenced by a number of

---

Box 3.6   Nuchal translucency screening – a lost opportunity?

Acting on 'intelligence' from a consumer advocate working in a major obstetric hospital, the independent New Zealand Guidelines Group (NZGG) proposed in mid-1999 that the NZHTA assess the effectiveness and cost-effectiveness of nuchal translucency (NT) screening for major chromosomal abnormalities. An emerging technology, NT screening at 12 weeks' gestation is becoming widely used in New Zealand, although it is not at present publicly funded. Feedback from women receiving the intervention suggested that they were receiving incomplete information on its risks, costs and benefits. There has also been a call in the UK for the procedure to be more rigorously assessed before it is widely used (Howe *et al.* 2000). Australia has moved recently to restrict access to publicly funded first trimester ultrasound scans largely for cost reasons.

The review suggestion was turned down for a variety of reasons, but principally on the grounds that it was not a priority as the procedure is not currently publicly funded. The NZGG thus commissioned a literature search on its own initiative to determine whether there is a place for best practice guidelines, at the very least to help improve the information that women are being given.

A year later, on 19 October 2000, a major newspaper, *The Dominion*, carried the headline 'Doctors warn of foetus test disaster'. This took place in an environment of high public concern about screening, following a public inquiry into cervical screening in a provincial city and concerns about a system failure in the breast screening programme in another city. There are now calls for the procedure to be publicly funded, with controls around the training of operators performing the scan.

Therefore, the debate is now about how to ensure that professionals performing the procedure are competent, rather than whether this is actually a worthwhile use of public funding in the first place.

---

factors, high-grade evidence for effectiveness and cost-effectiveness is increasingly considered to be a prerequisite. Information is also required to allow assessment against other important principles: equity, acceptability and likely impact on Maori health.

PHARMAC

PHARMAC has developed a clear process for considering requests from suppliers to list a new pharmaceutical on the Schedule (Figure 3.2). As for other decisions on pharmaceutical expenditure,

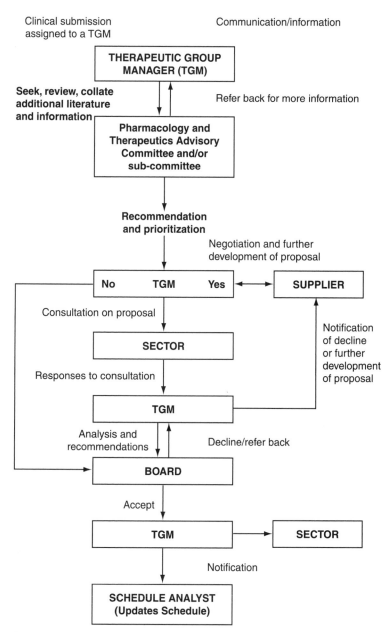

Figure 3.2 PHARMAC process for listing a new pharmaceutical on the Pharmaceutical Schedule

the assessment of new technologies takes account of 'needs, benefits, the impact on other areas of the health sector and the finite total health budget' (McNee 1999: 7).

In deciding which drugs should be partly or fully publicly funded, PHARMAC must balance evidence on effectiveness with cost. PHARMAC has developed considerable expertise in the process of cost–utility analysis as a way of comparing different drugs, both within and between classes, and deciding spending priorities (PHARMAC 1999b). The process used by PHARMAC is published and is considered a 'living document', to be updated in light of methodological advances and feedback.

When assessing costs, PHARMAC looks at both the direct costs of the drug and its effect on other parts of the health system. The process was applied in 1999 and 2000 in decisions to fund dorzolamide for glaucoma, tacrolimus for renal rescue and widening of access to lipid-lowering statins, as well as to determine access criteria for alendronate for osteoporosis and Paget's disease, beta interferon for multiple sclerosis, the widening of access to the atypical anti-psychotic olanzapine and the funding of lamivudine for chronic hepatitis B infection (PHARMAC 1999a, 2001). As information on drug efficacy is a prerequisite for registration, PHARMAC usually has good information on which to base its decisions. PHARMAC also receives expert medical input in making prioritization decisions from a Pharmacology and Therapeutic Advisory Committee.

It should be noted that drug registration is a separate process that is undertaken by Medsafe, a business unit of the Ministry of Health, whose principal concerns are with efficacy and safety. Interestingly, if a pharmaceutical company does not apply then a drug will not be registered for certain indications, even if there is good evidence for its efficacy. Thus, evidence based guidelines based on systematic review of international studies may end up recommending effective pharmaceuticals that are not actually available in New Zealand.

Overall, PHARMAC requires a high level of evidence (randomized controlled trials) for all its decisions and has developed considerable technical expertise in cost–utility assessment. The weight of evidence must demonstrate significant and cost-effective health gain. Other decision criteria help ensure that a high standard of proof is required before funding is agreed, including:

- the health needs of all eligible New Zealanders;
- the particular health needs of Maori and Pacific peoples;

- the availability and suitability of existing medicines or related products;
- the clinical benefits and risks;
- the budgetary impact, in terms of the pharmaceutical budget and the government's overall health budget; and
- the direct cost to health service users.

PHARMAC decisions can be appealed against by affected groups, who can reapply formally for listing. However, many people believe that such appeals, which are dealt with through internal processes, are largely fruitless as experience suggests that decisions are rarely overturned.

Failing the internal process, pharmaceutical companies have resorted to litigation. Over the past five years some $NZ4.2 million (£1.2 million) has been spent by PHARMAC on costs associated with litigation – about 18 per cent of operating costs (PHARMAC 2001). That PHARMAC has a near-perfect record of success in nine cases brought by the industry, one of which went as far as the Privy Council, suggests that the decision making processes it uses are sufficiently rigorous to stand close scrutiny. In 2001 PHARMAC lost its first case, which related to a challenge by PHARMAC to the decision of the Commissioner of Patents to grant patent protection for second medical use.

New technology assessment by private insurers

There are a number of private health insurers in New Zealand, which are playing an increasing role in the funding of health care, especially elective surgery. While Vote:Health[5] funding dropped by 11.4 per cent between 1989 and 1999, health insurance expenditure increased by 158.3 per cent during the same period. That said, health insurance still accounts for only 6.3 per cent of total health expenditure (Ministry of Health 2002). One company, Southern Cross, has over 70 per cent of the market share.

The issue of new technology assessment was discussed with representatives of the health insurers at the October 2000 meeting of the insurers' umbrella organization, the Health Funds Association. There was general agreement on a number of points:

- Needs are paramount in decisions about publicly funded services, while private funders are responsive to the wants of their customers.

- The introduction of new technologies by private funders is largely driven by the medical profession.
- There is great pressure to fund interventions that are not publicly funded, including those specifically excluded due to cost.
- None of the insurers has a well-developed formal process for assessing requests to fund new technologies, and some insurers have no process at all.
- Where a process does exist, the most identifiable part is 'clinical review', and most insurers rely heavily on the judgement of medical advisers.
- Informal processes play an important role – for example, 'checking' with other insurers as to whether they fund a particular technology.
- Explicit evidence for efficacy is seldom sought and some procedures are funded even when the evidence is known to be limited or lacking.
- Traditionally, health insurance was 'sold on choice' and cost was not a driver of decisions about funding new technologies, but this is changing.

Some of the comments were particularly revealing (see Box 3.7). There was considerable enthusiasm for co-operating with the publicly funded sector on initiatives to improve access to important information and the processes of decision making. However, a potential barrier to this was also raised: efforts to collaborate are

---

Box 3.7   How do private health insurers assess new technologies in New Zealand?

Usually, if someone [doctor or consumer] requests new procedure to be funded, I look around to see if any of our competitors are funding it. If they are, we invariably fund it because we have to remain competitive.

Essentially, we are at their [the doctors'] mercy.

The usual prompt for a request [to fund a new technology] is that the doctor has just attended an international conference, has learnt of it there and wants to try it out here – or be the first to use it here.

New technologies can give a competitive edge . . . will this help us sell [insurance] to the punters?

The private sector is at the 'sharp end' of the introduction of new technologies because of private surgeons.

often viewed unfavourably by the Commerce Commission as potential 'collusion' and anti-competitive.

Part of the problem for private health insurers is that the wording of many insurance policies does not provide many grounds for refusing to fund new technology, unless the intervention or treatment can be said to fall within one of the usually excluded treatments such as cosmetic or fertility treatments. An interesting example of where insurers reversed an earlier decision to fund a new technology is corrective laser eye surgery. Anecdotal evidence suggests that most insurers covered this procedure only reluctantly after one insurer offered coverage. It quickly became apparent that there was large demand for such surgery. This sudden demand led to all insurers moving to exclude this procedure from their schedules on the grounds that the surgery was largely cosmetic.

In summary, when making decisions about whether or not to fund new technologies, private health insurers in New Zealand rely heavily on the clinical judgement of the medical profession and on what competitors are doing in the marketplace. Evidence for efficacy and cost-effectiveness is seldom explicitly sought. Thus, the 'standard of proof' required is confined largely to the professional opinion of the doctor recommending the intervention. Appeals processes are internal and specific to the different organizations. Generally, appeals largely depend on the weight of consumer demand and clinician advocacy. If large numbers of customers want a specific treatment, then this is often sufficient to persuade an insurer to fund it.

CONCLUSION: HOW WELL DOES NEW ZEALAND ASSESS NEW HEALTH TECHNOLOGIES?

A number of organizations, both public and private, make decisions in New Zealand about the funding of health services generally and new technologies in particular. In the public sector, the principal decision maker has changed over recent years. Until December 2000 it was the national HFA, with some decisions made by the Ministry of Health. Upon absorbing the functions of the HFA, the Ministry became the key decision maker on funding; this function is now devolving gradually to the 21 DHBs. PHARMAC is the principal decision making agency regarding pharmaceutical expenditure. The NHC has a key advisory role in funding decisions.

Does New Zealand experience suggest the need for better information or stronger institutions for priority setting, including decisions about the funding of new technologies? There is clear evidence that both are needed. However, the general impression is that efforts to improve the quality of information – through initiatives such as the Cochrane Collaboration and the INAHTA – are outstripping the knowledge of many decision makers on how to access and use this information. This suggests that improving the processes for assessing and diffusing new technologies is currently more important. Even then, proper use of information is insufficient on its own to ensure that decisions will be well informed, transparent and fair. The examples demonstrate the complexity of decision making around new technologies, and that a principle-based and technically systematic approach is probably necessary but not sufficient.

In terms of improving the rigour and clarity of decisions, there are success stories. PHARMAC is arguably one such success, although not everybody would agree on this. In addition, a number of efforts have been made to help shift the culture towards one where examination of the evidence for cost-effectiveness is considered a legitimate part of clinical decision making. The NHC's guidelines programme was predicated in part on the notion that the whole health system is the sum of a myriad of individual clinical decisions. Changing the culture around the way routine clinical decisions are made should also influence attitudes towards introducing new technologies. However, such efforts are about long-term change and still meet with strong resistance; long-term investment in training is required if any culture change is to become embedded.

Whether or not New Zealand needs stronger institutions to improve decision making about new technologies, one thing is sure – the country has new institutions! The new structure presents both risks and opportunities. There is a danger that the expertise accumulated by the HFA in improving prioritization processes will be diffused by the changes and that considerable momentum will be lost. Smaller DHBs may not have people with the skills and experience to apply and further develop prioritization processes.

The changes also present an opportunity to consider what can be done to both strengthen prioritization processes in 'surviving' institutions and embed rigorous processes within new ones. There is a general need to improve the transparency of decision making processes and the new sector structure should assist this. Greater public involvement and accountability will require the DHBs to have clear and well-documented processes for making decisions about, *inter alia*, whether or not to fund new technologies. More formal processes to challenge or appeal against decisions will be needed to help DHB board members deal with the lobbying that is likely from local interest groups. Better understanding is also needed of the processes occurring at the provider level that generate pressure to introduce new technologies and of the way in which new technologies 'diffuse' through both the publicly and privately funded sectors.

Recent high-profile cases of quality failure have focused attention on quality issues more broadly. The introduction of new technologies in a timely, fair and safe manner is an important aspect of providing quality services. The principles that lie behind transparent and efficient introduction of new technologies are important dimensions of quality – effectiveness, efficiency, appropriateness and equity. Thus, the current focus on quality and concerns about the potential for greater variation in access to new technologies with the move to 21 DHBs provide a receptive environment for improving the processes of new technology assessment.

A proposal has already been made to integrate the activities of the New Zealand Health Technology Assessment, the New Zealand Guidelines Groups and Cochrane Collaboration activities in New Zealand. These activities, which have similar underlying philosophies, language and goals, could together provide a resource for the emerging DHBs for prioritization decisions and the assessment of new technologies. All three are committed to being a part of a broad culture change towards improved health outcomes for the population and high-quality health services, which resonates well with the New Zealand Health Strategy that will drive DHB priorities.

Finally, how does New Zealand stack up with respect to Daniels and Sabin's (1998) 'accountability for reasonableness' for decisions about new technologies? The publicly funded sector performs adequately (Table 3.2). Decisions are publicly visible and available on request, and most institutions demand the presentation of high-quality evidence to inform decisions. The HFA, until recently the principal funder, adopted a clear process for assessing new health technologies that is combined with a set of broad prioritization principles. These processes have been passed on to the Ministry of Health and DHBs.

Clearly, there is room for progress among private funders of health care, which they themselves recognize. Efforts to improve decision making processes cannot afford to neglect private funders, which are driven by fundamentally different imperatives from the publicly funded sector and rely more heavily on the professional judgement

Table 3.2 New Zealand's performance against the four accountability for reasonableness conditions in the introduction of new health technologies

	Publicly funded	*Privately funded*
Publicity	HFA/Ministry and PHARMAC decisions and rationales publicly available.	Unclear, but probably varies. Some insurers exclude specific procedures, and this information is available to prospective customers.
Relevance	Most institutions have explicit processes for identifying and considering both published evidence and the views of relevant stakeholders. The HFA (while it was the principal service funder) developed explicit principles, although these have not been publicly consulted on.	Evidence not often explicitly sought, and no clearly articulated principles. However, different imperatives operate, in particular retaining competitive edge. Medical profession dominates decision making.
Appeals	Internal processes exist, although most of these are not formalized. Ministerial lobbying occurs frequently and, in rare cases, the legal system is used to challenge decisions.	Unclear. Individual customers, sometimes with the support of clinicians, may challenge decisions with considerable persistence.
Enforcement	No.	No.

of the medical profession. Arguably, the private and public sectors should base decisions on the same efficacy and cost-effectiveness information, even if they may apply different values to this information, giving rise to different final decisions. By co-operating, private insurers gain a better understanding of the reasons why new technologies are not publicly funded, which will assist them to make their own decisions. Public funders benefit because, as in many other countries, most specialists practise in both sectors. Improving the rigour of decisions in the privately funded sector will heighten the expectations of both consumers and professionals of the 'standard of proof' required by both public and private funders.

NOTES

1   Ashley Bloomfield is an employee of the New Zealand Ministry of
    Health. The views expressed in this chapter are the author's own and do
    not necessarily represent the views or policies of the Ministry of Health.
2   The Core Services Committee was originally established in March 1992
    as the National Advisory Committee on Core Health and Disability
    Support Services. In 1996, the brief of the Committee was broadened to
    include advice on public health services, in addition to personal health
    and disability support services. The Committee's name changed at that
    time to the National Advisory Committee on Health and Disability, or
    National Health Committee.
3   For a fuller discussion of the role and work of the National Health
    Committee, see the Committee's annual reports, available on its website
    www.nhc.govt.nz (accessed 8 October 2002).
4   Since 1997, funding has been calculated by a Sustainable Funding
    Pathway formula, which takes into account predicted expenditure
    pressures from population changes, price increases, and changes in tech-
    nology and efficiency in order to maintain the existing level of services.
    New government initiatives are separately funded.
5   'Vote:Health' is the public funding for health and disability services that
    is 'voted' annually by parliament for this purpose.

4

CANADA
Douglas Martin and Peter Singer[1]

INTRODUCTION

The purpose of this chapter is to describe priority setting for health technologies in Canada. We begin by providing a brief overview of the Canadian health care system. Then we address seven policy questions related to priority setting for health technology assessment. Our overarching conclusion is that, although Canada provides a laboratory for innovation in priority setting, there is no mechanism to capture, analyse and share the learning from the various experiments in different contexts. Accountability for reasonableness offers a conceptual framework that could assist such policy learning and process improvement. This policy learning approach is probably also applicable to other jurisdictions, and offers an alternative to a more centralized approach as has been taken in other countries.

THE CANADIAN HEALTH CARE SYSTEM

'How do you describe the Canadian health care system?' is a trick question. In truth, there is no Canadian health care system. The Canadian health care 'arrangement' of provincial jurisdiction with federal funding and oversight was established by the British North America Act in 1867. Today's Canadian health care system evolved through a series of legislative initiatives (see Box 4.1). It consists of 13 independent provincial and territorial systems governed by their respective health ministries, with the federal government retaining control over health care services to specific groups, including the armed forces, prisoners and native Canadians.

Box 4.1   Key dates in Canadian health care policy

1867   The British North America Act establishes the basis for provincial responsibility for hospitals.

1947   Saskatchewan introduces Canada's first publicly funded universal hospital insurance programme.

1957   The federal Hospital Insurance and Diagnostic Services Act is passed. All provinces and territories are covered under the cost-sharing programme for hospital insurance by 1961.

1966   The federal Medical Care Act introduces federal/provincial and territorial cost-sharing for physician services outside hospitals. By 1971, all provinces were participating in the programme.

1974   A New Perspective on the Health of Canadians is released by the federal health minister. It reinforces the idea of broad determinants of health and calls for a reorientation of health care services toward health promotion.

1977   The Established Programmes Financing Act introduces a programme of federal transfers that are not directly tied to the costs of the provincial/territorial programmes.

1984   The Canada Health Act reinforces the basic principles which provinces and territories must meet to qualify for federal funding: public administration and operation, comprehensiveness, universality, portability and accessibility. It outlaws out-of-pocket charges for services covered under the act.

1996/97   The federal contribution to health and social services is consolidated into the Canada Health and Social Transfer, a major change in federal/provincial and territorial cost-sharing arrangements for health services.

Source: Canadian Institute for Health Information (2000: 7).

In 1984, the federal Parliament unanimously passed the Canada Health Act legislating five guiding principles (universality, accessibility, comprehensiveness, portability, public administration), and uses control over transfer payments it provides to the provinces as enforcement leverage. The Canada Health Act applies only to the physicians' services and hospital care available in each province. Ultimate priority setting authority in provincial health systems rests with the provincial Ministry of Health, although in some provinces much of the priority setting authority has been devolved to regional health authorities (RHAs). In all provinces and territories, priority setting also occurs within provincial disease management organizations, pharmaceutical benefit management organizations, hospitals and clinical programmes.

In the early 1990s, in order to eliminate its annual deficit, the federal government reduced transfer payments to the provinces for social programmes, including health care. These cuts forced the provinces to absorb the shortfall, which sparked a series of reforms, including the regionalization of health services, hospital mergers and closures, reductions in the number of hospital beds and average length of stay, reduced access to specialized care, and longer waiting times for non-emergency surgery (Canadian Institute for Health Information 2000: 8). As a result of these events, and extensive media coverage, public satisfaction with the health care system has plummeted in the past decade from 56 per cent to 20 per cent (Canadian Institute for Health Information 2000: 12). However, despite these 'crises', the health status of Canadians continues to improve – the infant mortality rate is 5.8 per 1000 births, and the life expectancy of Canadians is 79 years (second only to the Japanese) (Canadian Institute for Health Information 2000: 6).

In October 1994, the Prime Minister of Canada launched the National Forum on Health, a 'strategic planning' process involving consultations with academics, bureaucrats, administrators, health care professionals and the public. The Forum's purpose was to advise the federal government on innovative ways to improve the Canadian health care system. The Forum's two key recommendations involved the development of national pharmacare and home-care programmes – neither has been implemented.

In 1999, Canadian health care spending reached around $CAN95 billion – 9.3 per cent of gross domestic product. Approximately 69 per cent of health care spending is publicly funded; the remainder consists of private health insurance spending (e.g. prescription drug, dental and vision plans) and out-of-pocket spending (e.g. both prescription and non-prescription drugs). Hospital expenditures (32 per cent) consume the greatest portion of health care costs, and, since 1997, drug expenditures (15 per cent) have eclipsed physician expenditures (14 per cent) as the second highest health care cost (see Figure 4.1).

In order to rein in spending, provincial governments have been reluctant to approve the purchase of expensive health technologies. A recent study found that, of the 29 countries that belong to the Organization for Economic Cooperation and Development, Canada ranks in the bottom third on the availability of sophisticated technologies to physicians (Harriman *et al.* 1999). In September

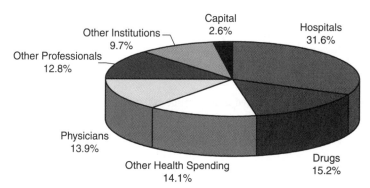

Figure 4.1 Percentage of total Canadian health care expenditures by use of funds (1999)

2000, in response to sometimes acrimoniously phrased demands by the provinces, the federal government agreed to increase funding for health and social programmes by $23.4 billion over the next five years.

Public examinations and discussions of the Canadian health care system are a national preoccupation. One national inquiry, by the Canadian Senate led by Senator Kirby, was completing its report in late 2001, and another, commissioned by the Prime Minister and led by former Saskatchewan Premier Romanow, was in full swing. In both inquiries, financial sustainability is a key issue. The current focus of the debate seems to be on financing and private sector involvement rather than learning from existing experience and organizational development in priority setting as proposed here.

EVALUATING THE CANADIAN EXPERIENCE

The primary purpose of examining the Canadian experience using the seven questions outlined in Chapter 1 of this book is to provide a fulsome description of how priority setting for health technologies is done in Canada. Unfortunately, we can forewarn the reader that the description below may fall short of expectations. It is impossible to fully describe how priority setting is done in Canada for three reasons: first, it occurs in a variety of contexts throughout the health system; second, a wide variety of methods, processes or techniques are used; and third, there are very few descriptions of what is actually done in these different contexts. We have therefore pieced together the Canadian experience to provide a general overview that does little justice to the individual initiatives that make up the experience.

What procedures are used to determine whether health technologies should be funded?

A key lesson from the Canadian context is that there is no single widely accepted procedural framework for priority setting. Consequently, priority setting occurs in various institutions using a variety of procedures, including formal technology assessments (e.g. by the Canadian Council on Health Technology Assessment), cost-effectiveness analysis (e.g. by provincial drug benefit management schemes), institutional committees (e.g. by Cancer Care Ontario (CCO)) and waiting-list management procedures (e.g. by the Western Canada Waiting List Project (WCWL)). Canada, therefore, makes a good laboratory for investigating different approaches.

In Canada, health technology assessment (HTA) is promoted as an important tool of priority setting for health technologies. However, formal HTA is seldom available for most technologies being considered. Important pioneering work on priority setting procedures has been done in Canada by Naylor and Hadhorn on waiting lists (Naylor *et al.* 1990, 1995; Hadhorn and Holmes 1997a, 1997b), and by Detsky on economic analysis (Detsky 1993). Yet since priority setting for health technologies in Canada occurs at various institutions in an unco-ordinated way, the procedures used by individuals and groups in different health care organizations vary widely and have not been systematically described, though a few descriptions are emerging (Deber *et al.* 1994; Giacomini 1999; Singer *et al.* 2000; Martin *et al.* 2001).

Below we provide a case example, the WCWL, in which we describe a concerted approach to priority setting on the part of a coalition of Western provinces. The case underlines the main point in this chapter: that there is a tremendous opportunity for learning from the decentralized Canadian experience, but that this potential learning is not systematically captured, analysed and shared.

Western Canada Waiting List Project

The Western Canada Waiting List Project (Western Canada Waiting List Project 2001), an initiative launched and funded by the federal

Health Minister in 1998, comprised representatives from the Canadian, British Columbia, Alberta and Saskatchewan medical associations, governments and RHAs. It consisted of five panels, which worked to produce a standard set of explicit criteria in the areas of magnetic resonance imaging, general surgery, cataract surgery, hip and knee surgery, and children's mental health. These criteria were developed into a specific 'urgency score' that would help determine the patient's relative status on the waiting list.

WCWL project panelists developed and tested the criteria-based scoring system in seven participating RHAs. In addition, they held focus groups with members of the public who supported the concept of a waiting-list scoring system as transparent and fair. Despite this support, research has suggested that clinicians who manage waiting lists have been reluctant to change their waiting-list management practices.

The WCWL project is an example of a priority setting procedure for health technologies in Canada. It demonstrates that a transparent and explicit process for developing priority setting criteria may still not be embraced by priority setting decision makers, in this case front-line clinicians, who have their own traditional implicit procedures. In other words, even well-developed substantive criteria must still be institutionalized, or used within the context of a priority setting process.

The WCWL procedure is one of many procedures used in various Canadian contexts, and important lessons can be learned from each. It is impossible to describe all these procedures because there has been no effort to systematically capture, analyse and share the learning from each of these contexts.

What is the role of different institutions in these procedures?

In Canada, institutions involved in priority setting for health technologies include: the federal government (e.g. the federal Ministry of Health established the WCWL project); provincial governments (e.g. the Ontario Ministry of Health determines funding levels for radiation oncology, and acts on recommendations of the Drug Quality and Therapeutics Committee (DQTC), the CCO and the Cardiac Care Network of Ontario (CCN)); the Quebec health ministry determines provincial funding strategies based partly on information from the Agence d'Évaluation des Technologies et de Modes d'Intervention en Santé; provincial pharmaceutical benefit management (e.g. DQTC); provincial disease management

organizations (e.g. CCN, CCO); RHAs; hospitals; and hospital programmes (e.g. a hospital radiation oncology programme (D'Souza
et al. 2001)). The complex interrelationship among these various
institutions in relation to priority setting has not been systematically
studied.

A particular Canadian innovation is 'regionalization by disease'
which has yielded provincial disease management organizations
such as the CCN. Consistent with findings from other countries
(Ham 1997; Coulter and Ham 2000), responsibility for priority setting is spread across all levels of the health care system, but
in contrast to other countries there is no national co-ordinating
body with authority to make priority setting decisions for health
technologies. Thus much of the decision making responsibility
has been shifted to institutional leaders, who in turn often diffuse
responsibility by establishing priority setting committees (e.g.
RHAs, hospitals, CCO and CCN).

This can be seen as both bad and good. Decentralization helps
politicians duck responsibility and avoid blame for tough choices
that may be unpopular. It may also leave complex priority setting
decisions in the hands of institutions and people poorly equipped
for the task. On the other hand, it allows leaders and stakeholders
at the front line, where decisions have the most significant impact,
to make priority setting decisions that best align with the goals of
their institution and best meet the needs of the patients they serve.
It also permits greater involvement by patients and the public,
who are more knowledgeable about the impact (i.e. on them) of the
priority setting decisions faced at the institutional level than they are
about decisions at a provincial or national level of the kind faced by
politicians.

HTA occurs in an unco-ordinated way in a variety of institutions.
Provincial (e.g. Agence d'Évaluation des Technologies et de Modes
d'Intervention en Santé) and national (e.g. Canadian Coordinating
Office for Health Technology Assessment (CCOHTA)) bodies have
been established to conduct HTA. Some of the institutions engaged
in HTA are listed in Box 4.2.

CCOHTA is a primary source of HTA in Canada. Its mandate
is:

> to encourage the appropriate use of health technology by
> influencing decision makers through the collection, analysis,
> creation and dissemination of information concerning the
> effectiveness and cost of technology and its impact on health . . .

Box 4.2 Some national and provincial organizations conducting health technology assessment in Canada

Canadian Coordinating Office for Health Technology Assessment (CCOHTA)
www.ccohta.ca/entry_e.html (accessed 3 October 2002)
Alberta Heritage Foundation for Medical Research (AHFMR)
www.ahfmr.ab.ca
British Columbia Office of Health Technology Assessment (BCOHTA)
www.chspr.ubc.ca/bcohta/
Agence d'Évaluation des Technologies et de Modes d'Intervention en Santé
www.formulaire.gouv.qc.ca/cgi/affiche_doc.cgi?dossier=3101&table=0& (accessed 3 October 2002)
Institute for Clinical Evaluative Sciences (ICES), Ontario
www.ices.on.ca
Manitoba Centre for Health Policy (MCHP)
www.umanitoba.ca/centres/mchp/1mchp.htm
McMaster University Health Information Research Unit (HIRU)
hiru.mcmaster.ca
Health Services Utilization and Research Commission of Saskatchewan (HSURC)
www.hsurc.sk.ca

[and] to facilitate information exchange, resource pooling and the coordination of priorities for health technology assessments. (www.ccohta.ca/ccohta_production/entry_e.html)

Although CCOHTA is a national organization, its reports merely inform priority setting in other health care organizations that conduct priority setting. One such organization is the CCN. The case study below features CCN and illustrates the innovation possible in Canadian organizations.

Cardiac surgery

Several parallel findings over the past decade have identified a need for examining priority setting for cardiac surgery in Canada. In 1993, one study showed that the overall rate of coronary artery bypass grafts (CABG) in Ontario rose by 31 per cent in the 1980s (Ugnat and Naylor 1993). Another study showed that waiting times from catheterization to coronary surgery varied among hospitals by as much as eight weeks, and over half of patients waited longer than the maximum suggested by an expert panel (Naylor *et al.* 1993).

CCN was founded in 1990 as an advisory body to the Ontario Ministry of Health mandated to improve quality, efficiency, access and equity in the delivery of cardiac services in Ontario. CCN includes all 16 hospitals in Ontario that perform adult cardiac catheterization, angioplasty or cardiac surgery. Its funding is provided by the Ministry of Health and Long-Term Care.

CCN engages in two main areas of activity:

- Coordinating the provision of advanced cardiac services for adults province-wide, with the aid of a computerized patient registry. This database is used by Regional Cardiac Care Coordinators in each cardiac centre to facilitate and monitor access to services by patients and their physicians.
- Advising the Ontario Ministry of Health and Long-Term Care on matters related to adult cardiac services. Using data- and consensus-driven methods, CCN offers planning advice for the future of cardiac services and the provision of high-quality care in collaboration with the Ministry and others.

(www.ccn.on.ca/mission.html)

CCN's patient registry has included cardiac surgery since 1990. In 2000, the registry was expanded to include cardiac catheterization, angioplasty and stent procedures. Extensive statistics on access to cardiac surgery are available on the CCN website. CCN makes priority setting recommendations, for example for the use of cardiac stents, to the Ministry of Health that the Ministry follows because CCN is in the best position to know what resources are required to meet the needs of the cardiac patient population.

What kinds of evidence do these institutions expect/require/consider in making funding decisions?

Although many different types of institutions engage in priority setting for health technologies, the evidence they consider is relatively similar and limited. There is a strong focus on evidence about effectiveness and cost, but a limited focus on other values that may be relevant to priority setting decisions.

Frameworks for legitimate and fair priority setting emphasize the importance of the rationales for particular priority setting decisions (Eddy 1994; Daniels and Sabin 1998). Priority setting rationales are important in both primarily private (e.g. US) and public (e.g. UK,

Canada) health care systems. In primarily public systems rationales are more often open to public deliberation, whereas in primarily private systems, where there is no democratic political mechanism for health care priority setting, rationales are often implicit (Daniels, personal communication, 2000).

HTA provides evidence for priority setting decision makers. As defined by CCOHTA, HTA is 'the evaluation of medical technologies – including procedures, equipment and drugs. An assessment requires an interdisciplinary approach which encompasses analysis of safety, cost, effectiveness, efficacy, ethics and quality of life measures' (Canadian Coordinating Office for Health Technology Assessment 1995: 2). HTA can be a bridge between research and policy making and is distinguished from effectiveness and health outcomes research by four key features (Battista and Hodge 1999):

1. Its focus is policy making.
2. Its content and processes are interdisciplinary.
3. It involves synthesizing existing data and, at times, generating new data.
4. Findings are disseminated widely and dissemination strategies are tailored to target audiences.

However, priority setting also incorporates other society-held values, such as legitimacy and accountability, and so Battista has suggested that we situate technology assessment within a framework of responsible stewardship of resources (Battista 1996).

Those engaged in priority setting for health technologies focus on published evidence of effectiveness (randomized control trials being the most valued type of support for evidence based medicine (EBM)), cost, and cost-effectiveness analysis (CEA), and make value judgements about the evidence. EBM and CEA represent the values of effectiveness and efficiency, key values in resource allocation decision making (Eddy 1996). However, these are not the only relevant values. Equity, public versus individual health, and the rule of rescue are some of the other important values in priority setting. These values could be redefined in CEA terms (Deber and Goel 1990; Eddy 1991), but perhaps a better way would be to go beyond EBM and CEA and incorporate these values directly in a synthesized approach, grounded in real experience and taking account of important values (Martin and Singer 2000). Moreover, formal CEA is not routinely available for many priority setting decisions regarding health technologies.

Although economic analysis (e.g. CEA) has also been promoted in

Canada as a more precise and apolitical means of resolving difficult priority setting problems, Canadian studies, like those elsewhere, have shown that economic analysis has a limited direct impact on actual priority setting (Battista *et al.* 1995; Holm 1998; Robinson 1999; PaussJensen *et al.* 2002). However, there is a increasing recognition of the importance of economic analyses which complements decision makers' growing desire for 'evidence' to support their decisions.

The first two case studies below, on low versus high osmolar contrast media and drug benefit formulary decisions, illustrate the focus on evidence of effectiveness, and particularly cost-effectiveness. The pharmaceutical case study is of particular interest because Ontario is one of the few jurisdictions in the world to formally require that manufacturers submit cost-effectiveness information. It illustrates the main point of this section that evidence of cost-effectiveness may be necessary but is insufficient, and has a limited impact on actual priority setting decisions. The third case, on priority setting for new cancer drugs, highlights the point that EBM and CEA are necessary but insufficient considerations when making priority setting decisions.

Low versus high osmolar contrast media

Contrast media are chemicals used in radiography that increase the contrast between structures of interest and background, thereby improving evaluation. Newly developed contrast media are lower in osmolarity than conventional media: osmolarity is the concentration of particles in solution which affects the movement of fluid in and out of cells. These new low osmolar contrast media (LOM) produce fewer adverse reactions than the old high osmolar contrast media (HOM), but cost considerably more.

Barrett *et al.* (1994) and Goel *et al.* (1989) conducted economic analyses of LOM and concluded that limiting the use of LOM to high-risk patients is justifiable as the incremental cost per quality-adjusted life year (QALY) in high-risk patients may be reasonable. The Agence d'Évaluation des Technologies et de Modes d'Intervention en Santé released a report evaluating the use of HOM versus LOM in Quebec hospitals (Conseil d'Évaluation des Technologies de la Santé 1990). The agency carefully analysed ten years of data on the use of contrast media and determined that the risk of death and other adverse events could be reduced by use of LOM. For example, they estimated that the risk of death could be reduced

from 35 to 27 per 100,000 with use of LOM in intracardiac administration of contrast, and the frequency of pain following injections
into a peripheral artery could be reduced from 66 to 33 per 100
administrations using LOM. The additional cost (for use in Quebec
hospitals, in 1990 Canadian dollars) would be $17 million per year
for parenteral use – $74,000 per severe reaction prevented – and $3
million per year for intracardiac use – $45,000 per severe reaction
prevented. They recommended that decisions about the use of
LOM or HOM should be made by individual institutions with input
from their staff and should be accompanied by guidelines for the
use of contrast media. Guidelines have been developed and implemented for use of LOM for high-risk patients, and outcomes
have been studied at some Canadian institutions and shown to be
acceptable (Barrett *et al.* 1998). There is now a trend towards
increased use of LOM.

Drug benefit formulary decisions

The Drug Quality and Therapeutics Committee advises the Ontario
Ministry of Health on what drugs should be listed on the provincial
formulary. Ontario's formulary is a listing of products the cost
of which the provincial government will cover for residents of the
province who are over age 65, are on welfare, or whose drug costs
represent a certain portion of their total income. Ontario spent
$1.5 billion in 1998 by covering costs for 2.15 million people (roughly
40 per cent of prescription drug spending in the province).

The DQTC recently adopted a published set of CEA guidelines
as an evidence standard for their analysis (Naylor *et al.* 1995). However, a study of their actual decision making revealed that economic
evidence had only limited influence on decision making (PaussJensen
et al. 2002). The DQTC does discuss economic issues, and occasion-
ally performs its own informal economic analyses, but these analyses
are usually used to justify decisions made on the basis of clinical
merit.

Priority setting for new cancer drugs

Over a three-year period, we studied the decision making of the
Cancer Care Ontario Policy Advisory Committee and focused on the
reasons it used in priority setting related to 14 drugs for eight diseases. A detailed description of the reasons is provided elsewhere
(Martin *et al.* 2001). In this section we will describe some of the key

lessons learned about evidence and reasons related to priority setting for health technologies.

Initially, the Committee members considered whether to develop evidence criteria that they would apply to each decision. However, finding that they were uncertain about the criteria, they decided to start making decisions and subsequently 'discover' the criteria. This strategic decision revealed that priority setting rationales involve clusters of factors. These factors included: benefit, harm, evidence, need, cost, availability of alternatives, precedent, convenience, budget constraints, total patient population affected, total cost to the system, access to treatment, pressure from physician and patient groups, and historical precedent.

Over time, these factor clusters were compared with previous factor clusters to ensure consistency (Jonsen and Toulmin 1988). Formal CEA was rarely available to this committee and not used. However, the concept was used informally. By observing actual decision making we learned that these factor clusters are a much more complex and nuanced form of 'evidence' than simple trade-offs (e.g. equity versus efficiency) which is the way priority setting decisions have often been portrayed (Bowling *et al.* 1993; Zweibel *et al.* 1993; Baron 1995; Nord *et al.* 1995; Ubel and Loewenstein 1995; Ubel *et al.* 1996a, 1996b).

Over the study period the committee twice requested budget increases, and both were granted. As the budget expanded, the range of considerations increased from, initially, only prolongation of survival and relief of symptoms to include reduction in toxicity and tumour shrinkage. Also, the committee initially vacillated about funding drugs that had only non-randomized evidence of benefit (i.e. phase II data), but eventually came to accept non-randomized evidence. This highlights the finding that, in the context of an expanding budget, rationales change. Rationales also change as costs increase. For example, the committee decided to fund an expensive drug for myeloma patients but not for patients with breast cancer. The evidence of benefit of the drug in the two diseases was very similar; the primary difference was the increased total cost related to the large number of breast cancer patients.

What standard of proof do they expect to be demonstrated in agreeing to funding?

Since there is no uniform process for priority setting in Canada, and no uniformity in evidence required by different groups, it will not come as a surprise that there is also no standard of proof for priority setting in Canada. Where such standards have been attempted, as with the Ontario drug benefit formulary example above, the application of the standard is hampered by the complex realities of actual priority setting decision making. Each institution pursues its own goals and uses context-specific processes to achieve them. To a varying degree, each institution relies on some form of published evidence to make priority setting decisions for health technologies. The standard of proof may vary, depending on the quality of the evidence. When the quality of evidence varies, institutions or groups must balance benefit against the quality of the evidence. An example of this arose in a CCN expert panel's analysis of intracoronary stents when they compared high-quality evidence of a small benefit of stent use for patients who had 'favourable coronary artery lesions', with lower-quality evidence of a potentially large benefit for patients who had 'unfavourable' lesions (Singer *et al.* 2000).

What appeals mechanisms are available for reviewing decisions?

To our knowledge, no institutions have formal appeals mechanisms available in relation to priority setting decisions for health technologies. In at least one instance, litigation has been used to challenge the findings of HTA, although the challenge failed. The pharmaceutical company Bristol-Myers Squibb Canada Inc. sought a court injunction preventing the release of a CCOHTA report on statins – drugs that lower blood cholesterol (Hemminki *et al.* 1999). The suit was unsuccessful and the decision, at least implicitly, protects the freedom of health technology analysts to publish their findings.

What does your experience say about the debate between those who argue for stronger institutions and those who argue for better information to support priority setting?

Both high-quality information and strong legitimate institutions are necessary to support priority setting. In regard to priority setting for health technologies in Canada, there are many organizations (e.g. CCOHTA) producing information (e.g. HTA), and an evolving, though less established, interest in strong institutions where the primary focus has been on developing committees with broad stakeholder representation (e.g. RHAs, CCO, CCN).

It is clear that in Canadian health care institutions the primary focus has been on developing information and information-related tools that can support priority setting decision making. These include evidence based analyses, CEA and waiting-list management tools. There has been some institution building (e.g. CCN), but this has been secondary to the information management aims. In general, there has been very little attention paid to the process of priority setting and organizational development in relation to priority setting; arguably, these are as important as information for improving priority setting (Singer 1997).

The National Forum on Health emphasized improved health information as a priority for evidence based decision making in regard to Canadian health policy. This is embodied in the Canadian Institute for Health Information (CIHI). The Forum acted as an advisory body to the federal government with the Prime Minister as chair, the federal Minister of Health as vice-chair, and 24 volunteer members representing professionals and consumers. One of the key findings of the Forum was that

> the health sector should . . . move rapidly toward the develop-ment of an evidence based health system, in which decisions are made by health care providers, administrators, policy makers, patients and the public on the basis of appropriate, balanced and high quality evidence [and] that a nationwide population health information system be established to support clinical, policy and health services decision making, as well as decision making by patients and the public at large.
>
> (National Forum on Health 1997)

Following, and partly as a result of, this report, the Canadian govern-ment committed significant resources to enhancing Canada's health information infrastructure, particularly through CIHI.

CIHI is an independent, pan-Canadian, not-for-profit organiza-tion working to improve the health of Canadians and the health care system by providing quality, reliable and timely health information. Its core functions are to identify and promote national health indicators; co-ordinate and promote the development and main-tenance of indicators; co-ordinate and promote the development and maintenance of national health information standards; develop and manage health databases and registries; conduct anlaysis and special studies and participate in research; publish reports and disseminate health information; and co-ordinate and conduct education sessions and conferences (http://secure.cihi.ca/cihiweb/dispPage.jsp?cw_page=profile_e).

To what extent does experience in your country meet the tests of 'accountability for reasonableness'?

A key goal for any group making priority setting decisions is legitimacy and fairness. Legitimacy – moral authority over priority setting decisions – requires an institution to have a legal mandate to set priorities and follow a fair process. Thus, legitimacy and fairness are distinct but related issues of justice (Daniels and Sabin 2002). Daniels and Sabin's (1998) four conditions for accountability for reasonableness are given in Chapter 1.

Recently, we conducted case studies of priority setting for new health technologies in two provincial disease-management organizations responsible for cancer (CCO) and cardiac (CCN) care (Singer *et al.* 2000). We selected these two cases because these institutions have tried to address directly the challenges of priority setting for health technologies, and because cancer and heart disease together are the leading causes of death in Canada. Our findings illustrate how groups facing priority setting for health technologies develop processes that correspond well to the conditions of accountability for reasonableness, but also face challenges not addressed by the framework.

Corresponding to the publicity condition, both groups identified transparency as a key element of a fair process and made their reasoning available in public documents. They also identified other aspects of their decision making that contributed to a fair process that accountability for reasonableness does not address – for example, acknowledging conflicts of interest, providing the opportunity for everyone to express views, ensuring that all committee members understand the deliberations, maintaining honesty, building consensus, ensuring availability of external expert consultation, ensuring appropriate agenda setting, maintaining effective chairing, and ensuring timeliness in making funding decisions to get effective new technologies to patients.

Corresponding to the relevance condition, both groups strove to make decisions that were based on reasons that the committee members considered relevant to their particular contexts. However, they found it prohibitively difficult to identify those reasons a priori and so found it necessary to start making decisions and then *discover* the reasons using hindsight. As noted earlier, the reasons they developed were based on complex clusters of factors including benefit, evidence, harm, cost, and pattern of death. Also, the committee members agreed that another important element of fairness was that multiple stakeholders were involved, including lay members (i.e. patients and community representatives). The groups discovered that a critical mass of lay members was necessary to facilitate their participation in the face of a potentially overpowering group of clinicians and other experts (Martin *et al.* 2002).

Corresponding to the appeals conditions, both groups agreed that a process for facilitating appeals was important. However, they struggled with how to do it effectively, and did not develop a formal appeals mechanism.

Corresponding to the enforcement condition, both committees were established by their parent organizations to make priority setting decisions using a fair process that was transparent and involved multiple stakeholders. However, both committees found this mandate challenging. For example, the cardiac committee debated the distinction between making recommendations for clinical practice and for funding priorities, and the cancer committee decided to advocate increased funding if it found itself denying an effective treatment to patients because of funding limits.

The actual processes developed by these committees bear strong similarities to the conditions of accountability for reasonableness. This suggests that accountability for reasonableness would not be a foreign framework if adopted as a type of common language to describe, analyse and share learning on priority setting among different health care organizations in Canada. However, accountability for reasonableness does not address all the challenges faced by groups making these decisions. In order to address these gaps, it is necessary to study groups making these decisions so as to identify and describe these challenges and to devise strategies for addressing them.

ANALYSIS

In this section we will provide an evaluation of the overall experience of priority setting for health technologies in Canada using the conditions of accountability for reasonableness. Since there is no co-ordinated strategy for priority setting in Canada, and no one central agency (such as the National Institute for Clinical Excellence in the UK) upon which to focus, evaluating the Canadian experience is piecemeal at best. Moreover, since priority setting occurs at a variety of institutions at every level of the health system and very few of these contexts have been the focus of systematic empirical study, there are few existing descriptions upon which to base such an analysis.

Since accountability for reasonableness was developed in the context of health care organizations and its conditions apply specifically to institutions, this is a helpful framework for evaluating priority setting for health technologies in Canadian institutions. In this section, we make a first attempt to use accountability for reasonableness as an analytical framework for priority setting in Canadian health care organizations. We find its conditions serve as useful guides for this type of analysis, suggesting that accountability for reasonableness may serve as a useful framework for policy learning on priority setting in Canada.

Publicity

In Canadian institutions, rationales for priority setting decisions are seldom available to anyone other than the decision makers. In some contexts (e.g. disease management organizations, RHAs) patients and members of the public are involved in priority setting committees, but the committee deliberations and their decision rationales are not accessible to the wider public. Consequently, the media, patients and patient advisory groups are seldom aware of the complex difficulties faced by priority setting decision makers. Since priority setting rationales are not made publicly accessible, there is no opportunity for patients or members of the public to engage constructively with priority setting decision making, nor is there any sustained policy learning.

Relevance

In RHAs and disease management organizations, groups or committees make priority setting decisions for health technologies. They try to base their decisions on evidence and principles that are relevant to their specific context. They often involve or consult patients or members of the public. These groups may meet the relevance condition. In other contexts, such as governments (e.g. Ministry of Health), Pharmaceutical Benefit Management (PBM) programmes, hospitals and hospital programmes, a narrower range of participants (e.g. administrators, health care providers) are involved in priority setting; patients and members of the public are seldom involved or consulted. These groups do not meet the relevance condition.

Appeals

To our knowledge, no institutions in the Canadian health care system have formal appeals mechanisms for priority setting decisions related to health technologies. In hospital programmes, a 'second opinion' may be used in dispute resolution when services are denied patients; this may not be considered fair by some clinicians, patients or their families, especially when rationales are not accessible to them. As mentioned earlier, litigation has been unsuccessfully used to challenge HTA. At the level of governments, political pressure may be brought to bear on politicians responsible for priority setting in particular situations (e.g. chemotherapy for breast cancer, waiting lists for radiation treatment). However, it must be noted that, if priority setting rationales are not publicized, groups may be unable to challenge decisions. This may explain why some decision makers, especially those in government, do not publicize their rationales.

Enforcement

Since we have argued that the publicity condition is not met, the relevance condition is only sometimes met, and the appeals condition is not met, it follows that the enforcement condition is not met. However, since responsibility for priority setting for health technologies is spread across all levels of the Canadian health care system, it is difficult to pinpoint who should enforce these conditions in particular contexts. Overall, health care priority setting authority lies with provincial health ministries, and the primary accountability mechanisms for these governments are provincial elections. Although health is a big political issue in Canada, it is rare that specific priority setting decisions in a health ministry actually influence an election to a significant degree. Moreover, health ministries are usually held accountable for their decisions, not their processes. To date, provincial health ministries have not enforced the conditions of accountability for reasonableness in any context, including their own.

FUTURE DIRECTIONS IN CANADA

Key lessons can be gleaned from the Canadian experience of priority setting for health technologies (see Box 4.3). Improving priority setting for health technologies involves developing strategies that use

---

Box 4.3   Key lessons from the Canadian experience

- Many different procedures are used in different contexts, but there is no mechanism for systematically capturing, analysing and sharing the lessons learned in each experience.
- Heterogeneity between institutions involved in priority setting has advantages, but a particular institution's priority setting goals are often unstated or unclear. Moreover, there is no systematic attempt to capture the learning that occurs in various institutions, and no sharing of knowledge between institutions. Therefore, there is no ongoing policy learning regarding priority setting in health care institutions.
- Although evidence based medicine and cost-effectiveness analysis are promoted, priority setting decision makers more often focus on other types of 'evidence' – this can only be documented by studying actual priority setting.
- There is no standard of proof for priority setting in Canada. Each institution pursues its own goals and uses context-specific processes to achieve them.
- To our knowledge, no institutions have formal appeals mechanisms available in relation to priority setting decisions for health technologies.
- The dichotomy of 'more information' versus 'better institutions' may be a false one. Both high-quality information and strong legitimate institutions are necessary to support priority setting.
- Groups struggling with priority setting for health technologies often actually develop processes and make decisions that correspond well to the conditions of accountability for reasonableness.

---

these lessons. Priority setting for health technologies occurs at various institutions across Canada without central co-ordination. The strength of this arrangement lies in the context sensitivity of the decisions. Each institution can make decisions that are deemed to be 'best' for the population they serve. However, since there is no central co-ordination there is also no central accountability for decision making regarding health technologies. The following seven strategies could be helpful:

1. Careful examination of particular priority setting problems (e.g. case studies) can identify root causes (e.g. budgetary versus human resource management).

2. Institutions could state clearly their priority setting goals and use them to guide decision making.
3. Case studies can be used to capture and describe context-specific practices regarding priority setting, and these findings could contribute to ongoing policy learning.
4. Studies of priority setting can reveal the evidence that decision makers actually use.
5. Institutions could establish formal appeals mechanisms to deal constructively and openly with challenges to priority setting decisions – this would also contribute to ongoing policy learning.
6. Continued effort could be directed towards developing legitimate and fair institutions.
7. Accountability for reasonableness provides a framework that can help Canadian health care institutions achieve legitimacy and fairness in priority setting for health technologies.

However, accountability for reasonableness is generic. It is not attuned to the nuances of particular contexts. For example, the conventions and core values that shape priority setting in a hospital will differ from those in an RHA. Therefore, learning how to apply accountability for reasonableness in particular contexts is an important next step for Canadian health care institutions. This may be achieved by examining each of the contexts using case-study methodologies (Ham and McIver 2000; Singer *et al.* 2000; Martin *et al.* 2001) and then analysing the findings against the framework of accountability for reasonableness.

Overall, we conclude that Canada would benefit from an emphasis on organizational development in relation to priority setting, capturing learning about priority setting that occurs in different organizational contexts, developing a platform to share that learning among different organizations, and adopting accountability for reasonableness as an ethical framework against which these empirical experiences could be assessed using a common set of concepts. Such a platform could exploit Canada's leadership and experience in developing a national health infrastructure, similar to the Canadian Institute for Health Information, which focuses on quantitative health system performance measures. Our proposal is for an 'institutional clearing-house' or 'quality collaborative' that would facilitate cross-institutional learning, focusing on qualitative description, analysis and sharing of 'good practices'.

NOTE

1   This research was supported in part by grants from the Medical Research Council of Canada (no. MA-14675) and the Physicians' Services Incorporated Foundation of Ontario (no. 98-08). Peter Singer is supported by an Investigator award from the Canadian Institutes of Health Research.

5

THE UNITED KINGDOM[1]
Glenn Robert[2]

INTRODUCTION

The UK's National Health Service (NHS) is a publicly funded national health care system, free at the point of delivery, which had two fundamental objectives at its foundation in 1948: universal coverage and equity of access according to need. To simplify, access to care is mainly provided through primary care physicians – general practitioners (GPs) – who deal with the vast majority of patient contacts but are also able to refer patients to specialist services within hospitals. Community services provide support before and after hospital care.

Within this broad model the NHS has 'never provided for every conceivable need' (Howell 1992: 1) and, as in any fixed-budget health care system, priority setting has always taken place in the UK. For decades the priority setting debate was played out away from the attention of the public at large as the NHS has traditionally rationed health care implicitly through 'non-availability, primary care gatekeeping and waiting lists' (Heginbotham 1992: 32). Then in the mid-1990s the Child B case drew widespread public attention to the ethical and practical challenges of priority setting.[3] In particular, this case highlighted how concerns to use limited resources for the benefit of the whole population have to be weighed against the urge to respond to the needs of individuals (Ham 1999).

This chapter examines priority setting activities in the UK from the perspective of three groups of decision makers: clinicians, local commissioners of health care and national policy makers. Such activities are continually evolving, as demonstrated by the ongoing review and revision of the mechanisms employed by the National

Institute for Clinical Excellence (NICE) in England and Wales. The chapter then assesses how well priority setting activities at each of these three levels meet the 'accountability for reasonableness' criteria set by Daniels and Sabin (1998).

PRIORITY SETTING AT THE LOCAL LEVEL – CLINICIANS AND LOCAL COMMISSIONERS OF HEALTH CARE

In the 1990s most decisions about which services to fund, or (more critically) which not to fund, were made through discussions at the local level. The NHS reforms, and particularly the purchaser–provider split, brought more explicitness to the commissioning of services (Locock 2000). Key players in these discussions would often include relevant health authority managers and members, fundholding GPs, and clinicians and managers in NHS hospitals.

During that decade government policies emphasized the need to target NHS resources on services of proven benefit. Decision makers, at least theoretically, were expected to consider evidence on the likely effectiveness of (mainly) new procedures and therapies in conjunction with their cost, when making judgements on whether these should be supported locally. While this approach had the benefit of allowing decisions to be made within local budget constraints and reflecting local priorities, it also had the effect of causing variations in the provision of services and was undermined by a lack of local expertise in assessing technologies. Following the most recent reforms to the NHS, responsibility for these decisions has passed from health authorities to large consortia of GPs called primary care trusts (PCTs).

Under NHS legislation, GPs in the UK have traditionally been able to 'render to patients all necessary and appropriate personal medical services of the type usually provided by general medical practitioners'.[4] The development of PCTs with responsibility for commissioning health services means that GPs are both agents for their patients and stewards of the resources for the community of patients they serve, raising potential conflicts for individual practitioners (Ellis 1999). To date, the day-to-day resolution of this conflict – between what Sabin (1998) terms 'fidelity' and 'stewardship' – has remained an implicit process for GPs, although the issues it raises have been highlighted by explicit rationing 'advice' directed at individual practitioners by national policy makers.

In 1999, for example, GPs – while having an obligation, enshrined in legislation, to treat patients according to their clinical judgement and patients' needs – received a circular from the Secretary of State for Health proscribing a specific treatment for certain of their patients (Dewar 1999). The treatment in question was Viagra for erectile dysfunction, and the subsequent legal proceedings initiated by the manufacturer of the drug resulted in a ruling which has important implications for priority setting in the UK. The courts determined that while the Secretary of State may issue advice to doctors stating that it is highly undesirable that they prescribe a particular product for a particular type of patient, the final decision on whether to prescribe the treatment or not must rest with the doctor (assuming that the product has not been added, via a statutory process, to the 'limited list' of prohibited drugs – see below).

Thus, while the traditional independent 'patient advocacy' role of GPs is fiercely protected, and has been supported in various legal rulings which have emphasized the need for flexibility in issuing policy directives, there are a number of mechanisms by which policy makers can disseminate 'guidance' regarding the provision of specific treatments to GPs. Such mechanisms 'preserve the degree of discretion in the treatment of individual patients that . . . provides the basis for implicit rationing in health care' (Ham and Coulter 2001: 167).

As well as specific cases which highlight the role of GPs in implementing priorities, there was increasing interest in health authorities' rationing decisions in the 1990s (McIver *et al.* 2000). This is evidenced by the willingness of patients to challenge those health authorities which refused to provide funding for, in most cases, newer and more expensive treatments (Dodds-Smith 2000). McIver and Ham (2000) examined four individual cases where disagreements between patients and families on the one hand, and health authorities on the other, did occur and a fifth case in which a health authority questioned the treatment of a medical specialist. Two of these cases involved challenges to the health authorities' decisions through the courts.

In the cases where the challenge was against health authority refusals to fund treatment which had been recommended by specialist clinicians, the challenges were successful and the health authorities concerned changed their decisions, although with varying degrees of reluctance. In the single case where the family was challenging both the specialist and the health authority, the health authority did not change its decision and, as with the Child B case, treatment was undertaken in the private sector.

In some regions of the UK commissioners in health authorities and primary care were supported by 'development and evaluation committees' which were established to provide research knowledge about the effectiveness and cost-effectiveness of health care technologies (Stevens *et al.* 1995). These committees adopted the concept of a 'hierarchy of evidence' to inform their recommendations, with the strongest evidence deriving from randomized controlled trials, and they used cost per quality-adjusted life year (QALY) ratios as an integral part of their deliberations. Around the UK there are a small number of academic research groups with a primary responsibility to provide independent advice to health services on the value of health technologies.

There have been few evaluative studies of health authority purchasing, and commentators have noted that in the early to mid-1990s health authorities were mostly concerned with gaining the basic information required to establish contracts and contracting arrangements. In addition, there was very little central guidance as to how actual investment or disinvestment decisions should be made locally (Hope *et al.* 1998). Such realigning of priorities is an area left relatively untouched by public debate as the NHS is not organized to routinely change existing expenditure if a new priority area is established or a new technology becomes available (Dewar 1999).

Consequently, there has been little explicit questioning to date of how commissioning (and therefore priority setting) affects the population's health or the provision of health care by switching resources between services or health care providers (Mulligan 1998). The response of many health authorities to the challenge of implementing research findings locally was to focus on marginal areas of disinvestment and restrict or reduce spending on services of limited benefit (such as surgery for varicose veins and hernias) (McIver *et al.* 2000).[5] Such decisions were often made on an *ad hoc*, implicit basis and the majority of health authorities avoided explicit deliberations around more contentious topics which might have provoked more public disquiet (Rao 1998).

Some health authorities did use methods such as questionnaire surveys, focus groups, health panels and public meetings to increase public involvement (Ham and Coulter 2001). In some cases these methods were used to gather information about the public's views and values to inform decision making (Cookson and Dolan 1999; Worth 1999) or to stimulate greater public understanding of rationing. More commonly, however, the methods were adopted as part of an attempt to consult with the public rather than directly involving them in decisions about priorities, although lay representatives and members of patients' groups were often included in decision making groups.

An interview-based survey of eight health authorities in one region of England with regard to the local commissioning of heart disease services found that where priority setting techniques were used at all they were adopted in an unsystematic fashion (Robert and McIver 2001). That is to say, resources for heart disease services continued to be allocated almost entirely on a historical basis without any systematic consideration of priorities either between different heart disease services in primary, secondary and tertiary care or between services across different disease areas. Indeed, in the absence of any form of programme or disease area budgeting, none of the authorities was able to provide a total for how much of their budget went into heart disease compared with other disease areas. There are, however, examples of health authorities and hospitals which have been more explicit and proactive in making rationing decisions by, for example, establishing a priorities forum to provide advice on rationing decisions with the aim of providing a reasonable 'due process' for decision making (Hope *et al.* 1998).

More recently there have been a number of instances of expensive new drugs becoming available which have highlighted the differences in the approaches adopted by health authorities in the UK. For example, in October 2000 the Alzheimer's Society reported that more than 50 per cent of health authorities were refusing to fund cholinesterase inhibitors for Alzheimer's disease (Aricept, Exelon) and that of the 35,000 patients in Britain who would be suitable for such drugs only a few thousand were receiving them (Laurance 2000). Such public discrepancies in the geographical availability of new treatments in the late 1990s led to the introduction of more directive, 'top-down' mechanisms with the explicit aim of eliminating this so-called 'postcode prescribing'.

PRIORITY SETTING AT THE NATIONAL LEVEL – THE ESTABLISHMENT, STRUCTURE AND OPERATION OF NICE

As a number of other countries had already done, part of the UK government's response to the issues raised in the previous section was to strengthen the information base for priority setting decisions. In 1993 it established a national health technology assessment (HTA) programme, and then in 1994 the NHS Centre for Reviews and Dissemination (CRD). The role of the HTA programme is 'to ensure that high quality research information on the costs, effectiveness and broader impact of health technologies is produced in the most effective way for those who use, manage and provide care in the NHS' (www.ncchta.org/abouthta.htm (accessed 8 October 2002)). The findings of the research commissioned by the HTA programme are not, however, directly legally enforceable in terms of altering either an individual clinician's behaviour or the decisions of commissioners of health care. The CRD aims to provide the NHS with information on the effectiveness of treatments and the delivery and organization of health care by conducting systematic reviews, maintaining various databases and fulfilling various dissemination activities. Prior to the establishment of NICE a number of other quasi priority setting mechanisms were available to national policy makers in the UK.

The National Specialist Commissioning Advisory Group (NSCAG) manages the entry of a very limited number of highly specialized services into the NHS as a whole.[6] Since 1985 the government has also had the right to place restrictions upon prescribing through the use of a 'limited list' of drugs. European law subsequently intervened via a 1986 European Commission (EC) Communication which set out some ground rules relating to the provision of reasons and proper appeal rights. Then the 1989 Transparency Directive provided that any decision to exclude a product from coverage under a national health scheme must be based on a statement of reasons, using objective and verifiable criteria that had been published nationally and notified to the EC. In addition, the decisions and reasoning, including expert opinion upon which they were based, were to be made available and affected manufacturers were to be informed of the remedies available to them in law and the time allowed for pursuing these remedies.

European law does not, however, currently provide substantive assistance to patients demanding treatments under the NHS (Dodds-Smith 2000). Hence, when the government attempted to limit the prescribing of Viagra in the late 1990s the courts focused on the *process* of decision making, as they have done with legal judgements on health authority rationing decisions, stating that the government's guidance should be struck down 'if the Circular was intended to and has achieved the same effect as if Viagra were placed in schedule 11 (of the "limited list" regulations) and none of the safeguards of the procedural requirements have been followed' (cited in Dewar 1999: 148).

Following on from the emergence of HTA in the UK, the Child B case, and through the well-publicized debates regarding treatments such as Viagra and beta interferon for multiple sclerosis, the generally uncontrolled introduction of new and expensive health care technologies has become an important and high-profile issue for clinicians, health care managers, politicians and patient groups alike. These continuing debates ultimately led to the establishment of NICE.

The establishment of NICE

NICE was created as a special health authority in February 1999.[7] As subsequently set out in the Secretary of State's directions in April 1999, its objective is 'to appraise the clinical benefits and the costs of those interventions notified by the Secretary of State and the National Assembly of Wales and to make recommendations'. More specifically, NICE has consistently been described as having three broad functions (NHS Executive 1999a):

- to appraise new and existing health technologies;
- to develop and disseminate clinical guidelines;
- to oversee clinical audit and confidential inquiries.

NICE's chairman has elaborated on these functions and has also detailed the concerns that led to its creation (Rawlins 1999a). In evidence to the Parliamentary Select Committee on Health in February 1999 he commented that 'over the past few years with new technologies, new devices, new pharmaceuticals . . . appraisal . . . has been undertaken . . . by district health authorities each acting independently with little warning, no horizon scanning, but suddenly presented with a new technology' (House of Commons Select Committee on Health 1999: question 5).

This has led to postcode prescribing, which has 'appalled health professionals . . . and [is] bitterly resented by patients and their families' (Rawlins 1999b). The hope is that through NICE advice postcode prescribing 'should largely become a thing of the past' (Rawlins 1999a: 1079). The Institute's website (www.nice.org.uk/article.asp?a=266 (accessed 8 October 2002)) summarizes thus:

> there are unacceptable variations in the quality of care available for different patients in different parts of the country . . . The Government is determined that this shall change to provide a genuinely National Health Service with dependable high

standards of treatment everywhere. National guidance, based on reliable evidence, is an essential part of achieving this. NICE will help to clarify, both for patients and professionals, which treatments work best for which patients, and which do not.

One of the main functions of NICE therefore is to produce and issue high quality, evidence based guidelines on the appropriate use of particular interventions. NICE intends to provide information about how practice can be changed and will also develop implementation methodologies to help local clinicians.[8] In 1999 the chairman stated that while the appraisals have caused the greatest interest 'it is the clinical guidelines programme of NICE that in the long term offers the opportunity to make the greatest impact on public health' (Rawlins 1999b) and – in more recent interviews – has continued to identify guidelines as the 'area where we want to grow substantially' (Cowper 2002: 94).

The structure of NICE

The Board of NICE meets in public and consists of a chairman, seven non-executive members (who are appointed by the Secretary of State) and four office-holders, who must include a chief executive officer, finance director and clinical director. NICE also has an advisory Partners Council that is composed of stakeholders and includes representatives of the health professions, health service management, the health care industry and patient and carer organizations. The last of these groups represents 25 per cent of the total membership of the Partners Council.

In 2000/01 the Institute had an annual budget of £10.65 million and 28 full-time equivalent staff (NICE 2000a). An early document setting out detailed proposals for how the NICE appraisal process should work stated that it is expected to be 'mature' by 2002, by which time NICE will be aiming to perform appraisals on 30–50 technologies each year (NHS Executive 1999a). NICE's more recent corporate plan states that 'by 2003, we will be producing around 50 sets of new guidance each year and reviewing up to 50 previously issued sets . . . Initially, we will be commissioning around 18 guidelines per year' (NICE 2000a). Following publication of the NHS Plan in 2000, NICE's annual budget was increased by £2 million to enable it to complete 50 per cent more appraisals and disseminate 50 per cent more guidelines each year.

An Appraisal Committee is appointed by NICE, and standing

members were announced in September 1999 (NICE 1999b). Members of the Appraisal Committee are appointed for three years, and up to five specific experts may be co-opted for particular assessments. The remit of the Appraisal Committee is to advise the Board of the Institute on such matters on which the Board seeks guidance. In particular, this is to include 'the use, within the NHS, of any new or established health technology in relation to its clinical and cost effectiveness taking into account the interests of the service as a whole'. At the end of the appraisal process (which was initially confidential – see below) the Appraisal Committee produces a final appraisal determination (FAD) on which guidance to the NHS is based.

The operation of NICE

In August 1999, NICE issued interim guidance for patient/carer groups, health care professional groups and manufacturers on how assessments would be carried out (NICE 1999a). This interim guidance was subsequently revised and updated in March 2001 (NICE 2001a). Each of NICE's technology appraisals and subsequent guidance to the NHS is based on three categories of documentation:

- an assessment report comprising a systematic review of the available evidence and an economic analysis prepared either by a designated and independent research team or by NICE itself;
- submissions from manufacturers/sponsors;
- submissions from professional/specialist groups, patient/carer groups and trade associations.

Submissions made by manufacturers or others are evaluated by designated outside academic groups or an appraisal team at NICE which may seek additional information from manufacturers. The Appraisal Committee then prepares an assessment report and a draft provisional appraisal determination for consideration.

The Department of Health in England and the National Assembly for Wales provide brief justifications for the selection of technologies to be appraised. For example, one of the first technologies appraised by NICE was hip prostheses, as two studies in the national HTA programme concluded that there was no evidence of additional benefit from using more expensive prostheses. NICE aimed to advise the NHS on obtaining best value for money for patients without reducing the quality of patient care (NICE 1999c).

To the end of March 2002 the 39 technologies which NICE has appraised and issued guidance on comprise 28 pharmaceuticals, 6 devices, 4 surgical procedures and 1 diagnostic technology, but no health promotion interventions. This initial work programme has led to some criticism that NICE has focused too much on drugs and technological advances, to the exclusion of community based interventions (Burke 2002a; House of Commons Select Committee on Health 2002).

The guidance that NICE issues on each of the technologies it appraises may take a number of forms:

- Where clinical and cost effectiveness have been clearly shown, NICE may recommend routine use in all patients for whom the technology is appropriate.
- For technologies where clinical and cost effectiveness have only been demonstrated within certain patient categories, NICE may recommend that use be restricted to specific groups of patients. The guidance may also suggest that, during a defined period of use within the NHS, further research is undertaken to confirm clinical and cost effectiveness in wider patient populations.
- In some instances NICE may indicate that a technology should only be used in the context of appropriately designed clinical trials. This is likely to occur in situations where, although showing promise, the clinical and/or cost effectiveness of the technology has either to be confirmed or requires further definition.
- Where the evidence for clinical and cost effectiveness is inadequate or lacking, NICE may recommend that particular technologies are not adopted within the NHS.

NICE (1999d)

NICE GUIDANCE AND GUIDELINES TO DATE

In March 2002, as well as the 39 appraisals on which guidance had already been issued to clinicians and managers in the NHS, a further 38 appraisals were reported as being 'in progress'. Raftery (2001) reported that of the 22 appraisals completed by March 2001, three recommended against the adoption of the technology concerned (prophylactic removal of wisdom teeth, laparoscopic surgery for colorectal cancer and autologous cartilage transplantation for defects in knee joints). In the period between March 2001 and March 2002 no further appraisals led to a similar recommendation, meaning that only three (8 per cent) of the 39 technologies considered to date had been 'not recommended'. However, the recommendations in the vast majority of the remaining 36 appraisals were couched in terms of selected patient groups or as part of an overall treatment plan. For example, Cox II inhibitors were 'recommended in preference to standard treatment but only when there is a high risk of patients suffering gastrointestinal problems as a side-effect of treatment' (www.nice.org.uk/article.asp?a=18030 (accessed 8 October 2002)).

Central to the establishment of NICE in the UK is how to *inform* and *influence* health care professionals' behaviour. With regard to the dissemination of clinical guidelines, five sets had been completed by March 2002 – on topics such as diabetes, myocardial infarction, and pregnancy and childbirth – and the development of a further 31 guidelines was under way. Rawlins (1999a) accepts that even clinical guidelines which are 'based on a rigorous and systematic review of all the relevant data must necessarily carry an element of judgement in their interpretation that may not be universally shared' (cited by Loughlin 2000: 10). Government ministers have emphasized this:

> The intention is that the National Institute will issue authorita-tive guidance to health professionals ... NICE will pro-vide that information, but NICE has no power to determine what decision is taken in each individual case. If a drug or treatment were ruled out on the NHS, that could only be by the Government, and therefore by Ministers, as is the case at present.
>
> (Minister of Health 1999)

The chairman envisages 'NICE as being a development of the [research and development] initiative in having determined the best practices and then disseminating them out to health professionals generally' (House of Commons Select Committee on Health 1999: question 7). He has elaborated by stating that 'health professionals would be wise to record their reasons for non-compliance [with the Institute's output] in patient's medical records' (Rawlins 1999a: 1079) and, quoting St Paul, 'if anyone disobeys our instructions, mark him well, and have no dealings with him, until he is ashamed of himself. But, do not treat him as an enemy, but give him friendly advice as one of the family' (Rawlins 1999b: 7). Although there is clearly an expectation that NICE guidance will be implemented locally, it is not yet clear what will happen if local clinicians do not comply with the guidance (Rosen 1999). As yet 'the legal mechanisms by which the Government will enforce any decision that a treatment is insufficiently cost-effective for the NHS are not yet clear' (Harrison and Dowswell 2000: 93) but we do know that 'if, having read NICE guidance, Ministers concluded that it should be enforced by regulation, it must remain the responsibility of Ministers to take such a decision' (Minister of Health 1999).

Importantly, the functions of NICE are closely interlinked with those of the Commission for Health Improvement (CHI), another relatively new organization which began its initial clinical governance reviews in August 2000. The Secretary of State for Health has made it clear that he expects 'health service organizations systematically and consistently to take account of NICE's guidelines' and that 'the new Commission for Health Improvement will help ensure this happens' (as cited in Beecham 2000). Monitoring is to take place shortly after the publication of each NICE appraisal and then six months later to track progress of implementation. CHI will then incorporate successive NICE appraisals into its clinical governance monitoring (Ferriman 2000). The fact that NICE is in principle advisory only is very clear: 'although NICE doesn't override the responsibility of health care professionals to make appropriate decisions based on the circumstances of individual patients, health care professionals are expected to take our guidance fully into account when exercising their clinical judgement' (www.nice.org.uk/cat.asp?c=129 (accessed 8 October 2002), July 2001). Based on new statutory obligations from January 2002 onwards, PCTs in England (but not Wales) have had three months to provide funding for treatments recommended by NICE, although this may be extended when more time is needed to establish new services (Dent and Sadler 2002).

It has been claimed that while NICE's first 15 significant decisions 'saved' the NHS about £70 million, recommendations for wider use of some treatments has boosted NHS spending by at least £205 million (Timmins 2000a). Raftery (2001) suggests that the first 22 appraisals led to a net cost of implementing NICE guidance of approximately £200 million (less than 0.5 per cent of annual spending on the NHS). However, it is still too early to say whether the NHS is acting on the decisions of NICE or to make a definitive assessment of its impact; research is being commissioned to explore these issues further.

Some anecdotal evidence highlights the difficulties that may lie ahead. One primary care group of 70 GPs has been reported as 'rebelling' against NICE's guidance regarding zanamivir (Relenza) on the basis that it did not agree with the Institute's conclusions. In addition – and perhaps more pertinently – they 'were rebelling against the diktat from [NICE], which made them feel that their individual clinical responsibility was being eroded' (Boseley 2000). A cancer charity has highlighted that the Institute's advice on taxanes for breast and ovarian cancer are being 'ignored' by many health authorities, with more than 20 per cent unable to confirm that suitable breast cancer patients are being offered the option of treatment with taxanes and nearly 15 per cent unable to confirm that paclitaxel (Taxol) is being offered to suitable ovarian cancer patients (Ferriman 2000).

The following section assesses how well the activities described above at the various levels of the NHS meet Daniel and Sabin's (1998) four tests of 'accountability of reasonableness': publicity, relevance, appeals and enforcement.

ACCOUNTABILITY FOR REASONABLENESS

Publicity

GPs and health authorities did not generally meet this first condition in the 1990s as, at these local levels of decision making, rationing remained, more often than not, an implicit process. While some health authorities did use a variety of mechanisms to engage with the public and interest groups, many did not and there are few examples of the public at large being directly and explicitly informed of priority setting decisions.

At the national level, the agenda papers and minutes of all NICE Board meetings are publicly available and make clear that, ideally, 'NICE is committed to ensuring that its deliberations, conclusions, and [the] reasons for its advice are as transparent as possible'. Generally 'as far as practicable all evidence sources should be made available for inspection' (NICE 1999a, attachment to appendix G, para. 16). For example, following the fast track appraisal of Relenza, a summary of the evidence upon which NICE's determination was based was made available on the Institute's website.[9] Evidence to support later final appraisals has been made similarly available, including the assessment reports that are considered by the Appraisals Committee. These independent reports are available on the Institute's website and, in addition, are published by the UK's HTA programme.

Leaks surrounding the Institute's draft appraisals of Relenza, taxanes and beta interferon prompted NICE to 'review its consultation process' with the pharmaceutical industry and professional and patient groups (Timmins 2000b).[10] As a result the Institute decided in early 2001 to publish its provisional technology appraisals as well as final appraisal documents. This sought to overcome situations where the wider public had been left debating the Institute's interim recommendations without being able to see the evidence on which it was based (Eaton 2000; Timmins 2000b). Dillon (2002: 97) states that the publication of interim findings 'marks a major change in the appraisal process and one which we believe will promote a greater understanding of the way NICE arrives at its rulings'.

One aspect where NICE initially fell short of meeting the publicity condition relates to the selection of technologies which should be appraised. The irrefutable need to prioritize important new technologies for evaluation has been recognized by NICE: 'We are not going to be appraising every single new incoming technology, the numbers are so great that it would be impractical' (House of Commons Select Committee on Health 1999: question 12). Consequently, as only a few technologies will be subject to national evaluation and guidelines through NICE, it will be important to select those technologies from whose 'guided' introduction the NHS is most likely to benefit. This raises the question of who is involved in selecting which technologies are to be considered and the criteria that they use in making those selections.

An earlier circular from the NHS Executive (1999b) stated that possible topics for referral to NICE would be identified from two main sources:

1. Information on new health interventions is gathered and prioritized by the Horizon Scanning Centre at the University of Birmingham.
2. Possible topics for guidance on existing health interventions or areas of clinical practice have been identified in the course of work on National Service Frameworks, supplemented by additional proposals from regional offices.

The circular went on to state that NICE's future work programme (after 2000) would be informed by a revised process led by the NHS Coordinating Centre for Health Technology Assessment. This process would 'enable NHS bodies to submit proposals for topics which might be suitable either for research under the NHS [research and development] programme or for guidance from NICE'. The emphasis would be on clinical innovations or new technologies that could have significant clinical or cost impact on the NHS, and on existing technologies where there were 'unexplained' or 'unacceptable' variations in use or 'uncertainty about clinical effectiveness or cost-effectiveness'.

The 1999 interim guidance to manufacturers and sponsors (NICE 1999a) and the updated *Guide to the Technology Appraisal Process* (NICE 2001a: 3) stated that the Department of Health and Welsh Assembly will select technologies for appraisal on one or more of the following criteria:

- Is the technology likely to result in a significant health benefit, taken across the NHS as a whole, if given to all patients for whom it is indicated?
- Is the technology likely to result in a significant impact on other health related government policies (e.g. reduction in health inequalities)?
- Is the technology likely to have a significant impact on NHS resources (financial or other) if given to all patients for whom it is indicated?
- Is NICE likely to be able to add value by issuing national guidance? For instance, in the absence of such guidance is there likely to be significant controversy over the interpretation or significance of the available evidence on clinical and cost effectiveness?

Evidence to the Parliamentary Health Select Committee in early 2002 suggested that those involved with implementing NICE guidance locally would welcome more opportunities to be involved in the selection of the technologies to be appraised (Burke 2002b; House of Commons Select Committee on Health 2002). Similarly, the chief executive of NICE has recently stated that he would 'like to create more scope for NHS staff to propose either clinical guidelines or technology-appraisal topics' (Dillon 2002: 96).

Relevance

Debates on rationales for priority setting decisions have rarely been held at local levels in the UK and have hardly ever involved patients and the wider public in any rigorous fashion. In their study of five separate contested treatment decisions from the 1990s, McIver and Ham (2000) commented that while all of the authorities gave careful consideration to the choices with which they were confronted – including in some instances making use of explicit frameworks of values in arriving at decisions – the rationales for their decisions were not always clear or accessible. In one case the health authority concerned agreed on the following set of values to help determine their decision: appropriateness, effectiveness, responsiveness, equity and efficiency. In three of the cases a review of the evidence of effectiveness was instrumental in leading to changes to the original decision to deny treatment. However, McIver and Ham (2000) concluded that – overall – decision makers relied on their own interpretation of values rather than any systematic attempt to identify the population's attitudes and values in relation to priority setting. They suggested that, given the attention received by the Child B case, it might be expected that health authorities were improving decision making processes in this troublesome area but that while 'this has happened to some extent further progress is needed' (2000: 123).

At the national level, the August 1999 NICE guidance stated that the appraisal criteria against which data are to be submitted are:

- clinical effectiveness;
- cost-effectiveness;
- the wider NHS implications.

In this context clinical effectiveness encompasses 'actual or projected benefits' which may include 'reductions in morbidity or mortality, improved quality of life, or other measures of positive outcome'. In the consideration of costs, both direct and indirect costs (including costs to both the primary and secondary care sectors and to the personal social services) are said to be relevant. The wider costs and benefits (including allowing patients to return to gainful employment) may also be addressed. The guidance endorses the standard approaches of cost minimization, cost–utility, cost–benefit and cost-effectiveness.

Significantly, in December 1999 the government announced that the regulations governing NICE would be amended to require it, when carrying out its functions, to take account of the 'effective use of available resources'. This amendment would appear to have introduced the subjective issue of 'affordability' to NICE's deliberations. This can hardly be seen as an unexpected development, given the presence from the outset of three health economists on the Appraisal

Committee. Furthermore, at least in relation to drugs (which represent over 70 per cent of the technologies appraised by the Institute to March 2002), without consideration of costs NICE would have been in many ways replicating the work of the Medicines Controls Agency.

In Parliament, ministers have said that the change in the declared function of NICE by the Department of Health's lawyers was recommended in the light of the Viagra experience.[11] Thus 'NICE will sometimes be forced to reject a particular technology [despite its effectiveness in a clinical context] in the interests of the service as a whole' (Rawlins 1999a: 1082). In evidence to the Parliamentary Health Select Committee three years later the chairman of NICE made it clear that the Institute deals with clinical cost-effectiveness but not affordability, and was clear that this remained the role of central government (Burke 2002a; House of Commons Select Committee on Health 2002) – that is to say that NICE, in and by itself, is not a 'rationing body' (Cowper 2002: 92).

Reaction to NICE's early recommendation to the Secretary of State that the anti-flu drug Relenza should not be available on the NHS did not augur well for agreement on the 'evidence, reasons and principles' upon which NICE guidance will be based. The reasons for the recommendation were primarily centred on what the Institute determined to be a lack of evidence of clinical effectiveness.[12] The decision brought predictions from the chairman of GlaxoWellcome, the manufacturers of the drug, that 'if the government continues to make the environment antagonistic to the [pharmaceutical] industry then obviously it will start to move elsewhere [out of Britain]'. NICE's subsequent endorsement of Relenza, based on later evidence, led to more publicity, with some GPs fearing increased consultations (Browne 2000).

The Institute committed itself to reviewing its guidance relating to the data it expects manufacturers to supply after it had conducted its first appraisals, including one each from the four technology types (pharmaceuticals, medical devices, diagnostics and procedures). This process of updating its *Interim Guidance for Manufacturers and Sponsors* began in the first quarter of 2000 through a consultation process with key stakeholders including industry, professional and patient groups, and resulted in the updated guide being issued in March 2001.

As Daniels and Sabin (1998) point out, 'the relevance condition does not mean that all parties will agree with the specific decisions made'. Rather the important issue is that those making the decision and those affected by it accept that the grounds upon which it is made are relevant. If this is the case then 'even those who say that specific outcome is wrong must admit that it is a case of reasonable disagreement' (1998: 59). The two 'grounds' upon which NICE's guidance is based which have generated the most discussion have been (i) the appropriate weight that should be given to patients' views, and (ii) the use of cost-effectiveness information.

Patients' views

Before NICE there was 'no organization that combined professional views with input from the public in order to make clear and informed recommendations on the methods of determining health care priorities' (Royal College of Physicians 1995: 15–16). However, the means by which NICE's Appraisal Committee takes into account and appropriately balances patients' views against clinical evidence are not clear. This issue has been brought into sharp focus as this is the first time at a national level that patients' perceptions are publicly and explicitly being taken into account. The Institute's corporate plan states that:

> Some of these [patient] organizations have expressed the view that the Institute must prove itself genuine in its desire to work with patient groups. We understand the reasons for this. NICE is a new organization and much of what we are doing and the way we are doing it has not been attempted before. We and they will need to explore together first how to define the unique contribution of patient advocates in our work and then how best to receive it.
>
> (NICE 2000a: 10)

Such concerns have been borne out by experience with a number of patient groups complaining of what they perceive to be a lack of commitment to including the patient perspective in the appraisal process (Eaton 2000; Kmietowicz 2001). Despite such problems, NICE clearly sees patient organizations as having a 'major role' to play, and this is one area where improvements have been made over the first three years of the Institute's operation (Cowper 2002). For example, NICE published further guidance on its relationship with patient organizations in October 2000 and is planning to establish a 'Citizens Council'. Such a forum, modelled on those used by the King's Fund, will be used to make ethical decisions (Burke 2002a; House of Commons Select Committee on Health 2002) – 'we will

ask the man and woman in the street to help provide moral clues'
(Cowper 2002: 93) – and to 'advise the Institute on the social, ethical
and moral questions that arise from our work' (Dillon 2002: 97). A
'jury' of up to 30 members will meet for several days – in public –
and produce a report on issues such as if and how QALY comparisons should be modified to make them fairer to older people.

Cost-effectiveness information

Daniels and Sabin (1998) highlight the controversial issue of cost-
effectiveness comparisons involving treatments for different groups
of patients with different conditions. It was not originally clear
whether NICE would use QALY comparisons when issuing its
guidance to the NHS (Freemantle 2000). The Institute did not
present such calculations with regard to the first three technologies
on which it issued guidance, and the chairman commented around
that time that recommendations would have to be based on difficult
judgements which have 'no mathematical quantitative approach'
(Yamey 1999). The Association of the British Pharmaceutical
Industry (ABPI) has highlighted concerns surrounding the use of
early economic evaluations of new and emerging health care
technologies. The ABPI suggested that realistic health economic
evaluation cannot be made until a technology has been in widespread use for a number of years, and that delaying entry of some
technologies into the NHS could have a negative impact on health
care services and be 'a disservice to patients' (ABPI 1999).

NICE's more recently published corporate plan acknowledges
such concerns regarding the use of cost-effectiveness information
while committing the Institute to taking the issue into consideration
when issuing its guidance:

> Health professionals have also been confused by the need to
> balance clinical with cost effectiveness. Most (albeit, in some
> instances, reluctantly) accept that all health care systems have
> finite resources; and they seek to provide services which offer
> the best value for money for the population as a whole. Few
> independent evaluations of individual health technologies, and
> even fewer clinical guidelines, have been constructed to take
> account of these inter-related issues. The Institute's guidance
> will, invariably, be based on evidence of both clinical and cost
> effectiveness.
>
> (NICE 2000a: 3)

Such an acknowledgement does, at least tentatively, begin to hold the prospect of NICE having a broader public impact in terms of legitimizing cost-effectiveness criteria.

Approximately half of the guidance documents to be issued have incorporated cost per QALY figures (Raftery 2001). In addition, a number of the assessment reports considered by the Appraisals Committee have either presented such figures (while often commenting on their speculative nature) or recommended the need for further relevant research before such calculations can be made. In a review of NICE guidance to March 2001, Raftery (2001: 1302) could not 'conclusively establish how the balance between clinical benefit and economics (cost per QALY) influences NICE recommendations'.

This limited use of cost-effectiveness ratios may reflect the varying evidence bases for the different types of technology which NICE has appraised to date: data to calculate cost per QALY estimates are often more readily available for pharmaceuticals (i.e. taxanes) than procedures (i.e. wisdom teeth extraction) or devices (i.e. hip prostheses). In the latter cases the confidence intervals around any cost per QALY estimates which NICE might include in its guidance are likely to be very large.

Despite this, in mid-2001 it appeared that a QALY threshold was emerging from the deliberations of NICE. As cited by McDonald (2001), NICE agenda papers[13] stated: 'It would appear that the Appraisal Committee has been reluctant to recommend the use of technologies with a cost per-life-year gained, or QALY, of more than £30,000. In future, the Committee should provide very clear reasons for recommending technologies . . . where the . . . QALY is in excess of £30,000'. The chairman of NICE has subsequently denied that any simple threshold is applied, talking rather of a 'curve': the higher the cost of a technology, the more convincing the evidence for its use must be (Cowper 2002). For all types of technologies, however, the determination of what is an acceptable cost-effectiveness threshold, and what is not, is not simply a technical judgement but an ethical one (Smith 2000).

Appeals

McIver and Ham (2000) found that in only one of the five health authorities which they studied was there an appeals mechanism. Rather it appears that appeals against (often implicit) rationing decisions – which have been highlighted by well-publicized individual cases – have almost entirely been made through the legal system. Certainly the experience of a number of such cases in the 1990s has shown that appeals procedures within those NHS bodies making rationing decisions have been insufficient and not explicitly built into decision making processes.

In contrast, the appeals procedure following NICE's deliberations regarding a technology were outlined in July 1999 (NICE 1999a). Later guidance issued in June 2001 makes clear that an appeal may be made by the manufacturers, sponsors, patients' and carers' representative groups and appropriate professional bodies (NICE 2001b).

The specific grounds on which an appeal may be made, and will be heard, are as follows:

1. The Institute has failed to act fairly and in accordance with the Appraisal Procedure set out in the Institute's *Guide to the Technology Appraisal Process.*
2. The Institute has prepared guidance which is perverse in the light of the evidence submitted.
3. The Institute has exceeded its powers.

(NICE 2001b: 3)

The guidance explicitly states that:

An appeal is not an opportunity to reopen arguments and issues upon which the Appraisal Committee has reached a determination. The Appeal Panel will not substitute its own judgement for that of the Appraisal Committee or look afresh at the evidence submitted to the Appraisal Committee. The Appeal Panel has the restricted role of hearing appeals which fall within one or more of the three strictly limited grounds upon which interested parties may appeal. An appeal on any other ground will not be considered.

(NICE 2001b: 3).

The guidance to date does not therefore appear to contemplate a meaningful appeal on the merits of a recommendation but rather only submissions as to procedural fairness (unless the appeal is based on the contention that the decision is perverse) (Dodds-Smith 2000). Furthermore, only under 'exceptional circumstances' will NICE revise its decisions in the light of further evidence *prior to* the official review date for the guidance. In general, 'the Institute will not review any guidance earlier than twelve months after its original publication date' (NICE 2001a: 17).

However, given the reliance that NICE has had to place on modelling exercises (because of the paucity of data available about most new technologies at the time of its deliberations) it can 'expect to receive challenges from groups or individuals who disagree with [its] recommendations' (Coulter 1999). Indeed appeals were made, and rejected, against the determinations on both Relenza and hip prostheses (NICE 2000b). However, appeals against the guidance from NICE as it related to the use of paclitaxel in the second-line treatment of breast cancer were upheld in May 2000. The grounds for this decision were that the Institute failed to act fairly and in accordance with the Appraisal Procedure set out in the *Interim Guidance for Manufacturers and Sponsors*[14] and that the Institute had prepared guidance which was perverse in the light of the evidence submitted.[15]

Concerns have also been raised that 'the appraisal system could get bogged down if the need for an early reappraisal delays work on other emerging technologies' (Rosen 1999: 7). Currently the Institute issues a clear statement of when its guidance will be reviewed as each appraisal is published. So, for example, when guidance on the use of liquid-based cytology for cervical screening was issued in June 2000 it was accompanied by a statement that it would be reviewed in May 2002 or once the outcome of pilot studies (recommended in the guidance) is known (NICE 2000c).

Enforcement

McIver and Ham (2000) suggest that the challenges launched by patients and families and the involvement of lawyers and the courts were instrumental in forcing health authorities to review their policies and procedures, and that decision making arrangements were strengthened as a result. However, the regulation of this process was limited to legal oversight, and in the English courts this focuses mainly on the way in which decisions are made rather than their rationales – thus 'the NHS still lacks rigorous and consistent decision making processes for dealing with cases of this kind' (2000: 122).

As described above, NICE has a carefully constructed constitution and operating arrangements which are constantly under review. The regulation of NICE's processes for making decisions is examined – and its officers implicitly held to account for 'reasonableness' – by the Parliamentary Health Select Committee. The Select Committee comprises Members of Parliament drawn from across the political parties and is appointed to examine the 'expenditure, administration and policy of the Department of Health and associated public bodies' and has 'the power to send for persons, papers and records' (http://www.parliament.uk/commons/selcom/hlthhome.htm (accessed 8 October 2002)). NICE has been the subject of an inquiry by the Select Committee on two occasions. In early 2002 the Select Committee considered 'the progress NICE has made in achieving . . . key goals', namely that it:

- is providing clear and credible guidance
- has ended confusion by providing a single national focus
- is providing guidance that is locally owned and acted on in the right way
- is actively promoting interventions with good evidence of clinical and cost-effectiveness so that patients have faster access to treatments known to work (House of Commons Select Committee on Health 2002)

This particular inquiry also specifically sought to examine the independence of NICE. Submission of written evidence relating to these issues was publicly invited and oral evidence taken from a wide range of stakeholders including patient groups, charities, health authorities, pharmaceutical companies and academics, as well as senior officers from NICE itself. The final reports of such inquiries are freely available. Notwithstanding the periodic attentions of the Select Committee, ongoing enforcement of the first three criteria from the tests for 'accountability for reasonableness' remains essentially a voluntary process, reliant on the good intentions and integrity of those charged with fulfilling NICE's legislated tasks.

DISCUSSION

How far do current decision making processes meet the tests of 'accountability for reasonableness'?

The concept of 'accountability for reasonableness' is just as important in a tax-funded national health service as it was in its original application to managed care plans in the United States. Overall it aims to educate clinicians and patients about the need for limits and empowers a more focused public deliberation in which ultimate authority for limiting care rests with the democratic processes (Daniels and Sabin 1998).

With regard to current decision making processes relating to priority setting in the NHS, accountability for reasonableness is not generally fulfilled at the level of either the individual medical practitioner or local commissioners of health care. There is still relatively little direct publicity or debate regarding rationing decisions at the local level, few explicit sets of rationales are available, and appeals are, for the most part, settled by default through the courts. The latter have emphasized the need for such 'fair processes' in the handful of cases which have been heard in the UK (such directions also being supported indirectly by elements of the national and European law), but no single piece of comprehensive legislation exists to oversee the decision making process at these levels of the health care system in the UK.

In contrast, NICE certainly meets the 'publicity' condition in terms of ensuring that its decisions, and the evidence upon which those decisions are based, are made publicly and widely available. One relatively minor question remains concerning just how the technologies to be considered by NICE are selected. There is certainly some recognition of the lines of democratic accountability under which NICE operates as it 'ultimately has to temper its advice in relationship to the people's elected representatives in parliament and in Government' (House of Commons Select Committee on Health 1999, question 35). NICE also broadly meets the 'relevance' and 'appeals and revision of advice' conditions, although a number of important – and as yet unresolved – issues have been raised here in relation to these aspects. Finally, it is not yet clear how enforcement of the first three criteria will be applied to NICE's decision making processes beyond the expectation that it will be the subject of inquiries from the Health Select Committee on an ongoing basis.

One issue which merits further discussion is how formal rationing processes can meet Daniels and Sabin's criteria while avoiding unnecessary delays in the introduction of technologies which ultimately prove to be beneficial and cost-effective (Burke 2002c). NICE envisages being involved in promoting such technologies: 'by encouraging innovation and helping "ensure that when innovative products do become available they reach patients as quickly as possible"' (Rawlins 1999b). This has happened with regard to the introduction of rosiglitazone, a drug for type II diabetes, which the Institute is supporting: 'this guidance is an example of the way NICE intends to support and promote clinically and cost effective new medicines at the time they become available. Our guidance should ensure uniform take up of rosiglitazone throughout the NHS' (NICE 2000b).

In the future the achievement of this aim should be greatly assisted by the availability of earlier warning well in advance of the new technology being launched or introduced to the NHS, but this will be reliant to a large extent on a good working relationship with manufacturers and pharmaceutical companies in particular.

Role of information and institutions

There has been a clear attempt in the UK to improve the evidence base for making priority setting decisions through a number of national initiatives (e.g. through the ongoing support for the HTA programme and the CRD). However, improving the information base alone is insufficient. While this may plug some of the gaps in existing knowledge and supplement a culture of evidence based medicine, differences in the interpretation of research evidence will remain: lengthy delays in NICE reaching a final decision regarding beta interferon were due in large part to 'serious reservations' about the economic models used and, in particular, to doubts regarding some of the assumptions made in those models (NICE 2001c; Sculpher *et al.* 2001).

The introduction of agencies such as NICE is a clear example of the concern to strengthen the institutional basis of rationing (Ham and Coulter 2001). Indeed, NICE could be seen as entailing a move away from an 'old' model which focused on providing information regarding new technologies and incentives to a 'new' model which involves a formal mechanism for a centralized decision or recommendation (Buxton 1999). NICE also accepts that manufacturers may not be able to provide full information of the type required to make an optimal evaluation. The chairman of NICE believes that

> many of these things can be resolved if the economic aspects are included in the clinical trials starting way back ... as NICE becomes more mature and as the industry becomes more accepting of the need for this sort of additional data-gathering ... this issue will be relatively resolvable.
>
> (House of Commons Select Committee on Health 1999:
> question 30)

In at least the medium term this must remain a somewhat optimistic hope and raises, not least, some important methodological issues which have been touched on by, among others, the ABPI. In particular, it will be harder to obtain data for non-drug technologies which at present do not have to undergo as rigorous a scrutiny as new drugs before they are introduced to the NHS (Coulter 1999). Similarly, requests for a more open collaboration with manufacturers also appear to be based rather more on hope than expectation as borne out by evidence taken by the Health Select Committee in early 2002 (Burke 2002a).

When the required evidence has not become available at the point that a product comes to market, NICE envisages recommending that in the first instance the NHS channels the use of the new technology through well-controlled research studies. For example, NICE finally announced its decision regarding beta interferon in early 2002 after a lengthy and contentious period of consultation (NICE 2001c) much of which was conducted under high levels of public interest and scrutiny. While recommending against the use of beta interferon by the NHS, NICE and five pharmaceutical manufacturers united in favour of a 'payment by results' scheme. Under the scheme, eligible patients will undergo a lengthy assessment of their baseline level of disability against which the disease progression and treatment effect will be compared each year for ten years. The NHS will fund treatment until it is deemed to be no longer effective. Costs to the NHS will be adjusted according to whether expected benefits to patients are realized; the price of the drug will drop if expected clinical improvement targets are not met. The expected annual NHS bill is estimated at £50 million (Little 2002).

In order to avoid ineffective investment in improving the information base for decisions, research prioritization (such as that undertaken in the case of beta interferon) must take direct account of the real health care policy-making environment, linking the likelihood that research will in practice influence decisions in a 'rational' way to specific outcomes of the research. Policy makers and NICE will require analyses that consider both the theoretical value of information and the likely behavioural response to it. Analysis of the value of information may offer a way to improve our estimates of the former; better political science based understanding of what influences policy making may help to underpin our estimates of the latter. In summary, 'the choice available to policy makers is not between more information and stronger institutions, rather it is how the work of institutions can be enhanced through the provision of better information and other mechanisms' (Ham and Coulter 2001: 166).

CONCLUSIONS

Few would argue against the principles which lie behind the establishment of NICE, and it appears to broadly meet all of the requirements of accountability for reasonableness. However, the successful application of these principles will require a more open and honest debate about the state of the NHS and its ability to respond to all the demands which are being placed upon it now and will be placed upon it in the future. As Daniels and Sabin (1998: 61) state, their four conditions 'provide connective tissue to, not a replacement for, a broader democratic process'. NICE itself has sometimes seemingly backed off from controversy, which must go some way to explaining – at least in part – the lengthy process before a decision was reached on beta interferon for multiple sclerosis (Mayor 2001; NICE 2001c; Little 2002).

One of the biggest remaining questions in the UK, and the issue which will be the key to the success or otherwise of NICE, concerns the Institute's ability to disseminate its guidance effectively to those who are faced with priority setting dilemmas on an almost daily basis: the health care professionals who care for and treat patients in the NHS. This is not to say that this vital issue has gone unrecognized, for over the first three years of its operation NICE has acknowledged that it has to become more 'subtle and facilitative' in order for implementation of its recommendations to take place locally and that the Institute 'could [have done] more to help this process' (Cowper 2002: 92). Nonetheless, pending the findings of research commissioned by NICE, the jury is still out on how success-fully its guidance is disseminated and implemented in the NHS.

One clear problem for local commissioners of health care in this regard is that NICE does not routinely provide comparative infor-mation either on the cost-effectiveness of the various technologies for which it issues guidance or on any potential alternative treat-ments or services (Cookson *et al.* 2001). By providing judgements which relate solely to individual technologies – and expecting these to be implemented – NICE guidance can leave local commissioners with the difficult problem of having to fund the technologies in question even though, in some cases, these may be less cost-effective than other existing treatments and services.

As a consequence, one possible scenario is that, alongside the 'fair' processes established by NICE, individual PCTs may make different decisions as to local priorities. This outcome may be difficult to accept in a publicly funded health care system but – if all involved have used 'fair' processes for deliberation – reasonable people may still disagree (Daniels and Sabin 1998) and so policy makers may have to accept that local commissioning decisions may still vary. The implication of this is that attempts to eradicate 'post-code prescribing', one of the *raisons d'être* of NICE, may ultimately still fail.

Daniels and Sabin (1998: 64) suggest that 'establishing the accountability of decision makers to those affected by their decisions is the only way to show, over time, that arguably fair decisions are being made and that those making them have established a procedure we should view as legitimate'. In relation to the degree of support that the broader public will give to the emerging work of NICE (Lenaghan 1999), the chairman of NICE has stated that, 'perhaps most important of all, [NICE needs] to earn and retain the confidence of patients and the public, health professionals and managers, and the health care industry' (Rawlins 1999b). And yet he has also repeatedly stated that he does not 'see a role for the Institute in the rationing of treatments to NHS patients' (Rawlins 1999b), preferring to couch the debate in terms of 'prioritisation' (Rawlins 1999a: 1082). Commentators have seen this 'failure of honesty' as possibly leading to the ultimate failure of NICE (Smith 2000: 1364).

In spite of recent institutional developments with regard to priority setting in the UK – developments which have complemented an already strong emphasis on evidence based decision making – there remains a need for a more open and honest public debate regarding the inevitable need for rationing of scarce health care resources and the best processes by which to achieve this. Although NICE's task is sometimes seen as a 'mission impossible' (Dillon 2002: 96), by partaking more explicitly in this debate – and through its still emergent working processes – it may still make a wider and longer lasting contribution to health care priority setting in the UK.

NOTES

1 NICE produces guidance for the NHS in England and Wales. The Health Technology Board for Scotland (technology appraisals) and Scottish Intercollegiate Guidelines Network (clinical guidelines) develop guidance for the NHS in Scotland but 'wherever possible, it [NICE] collaborates closely on work programmes with its Scottish counterparts' (www.nice.org.uk/cat.asp?c=32252 (accessed 8 October 2002), May 2002). See Cookson *et al.* (2001) and subsequent electronic responses

(http://bmj.com.cgi/eletters/323/7315/743) for further discussion of priority setting arrangements in Scotland.

2 The author is grateful to Mr Andrew Dillon, chief executive of NICE, and to Professor Andrew Stevens, Professor of Public Health and Epidemiology, University of Birmingham and member of the NICE appraisal committee, for comments in late 2000 on an early draft of this chapter.

3 Child B was diagnosed as having non-Hodgkin's lymphoma and then a second cancer, acute myeloid leukaemia. The paediatricians responsible for her care advised that she had 6–8 weeks to live. Their view was that the child's medical history meant she was unlikely to benefit from further intensive treatment, and they recommended palliative care. The child's father eventually sought leave for judicial review to challenge the health authority decision not to fund treatment at a second hospital which was prepared to consider a second bone marrow transplant at an estimated cost of £75,000. This was granted. The High Court took the view that the right to life was so precious that the health authority should reconsider its decision, even though the chances of success were acknowledged to be low. This judgment was overturned on appeal.

4 From the statutory terms of service as set out in Schedule 2 to the NHS (General Medical Services) Regulations 1992 and as cited in Dodds-Smith (2000).

5 Klein and Redmayne reported how in 1996/97, 26 of 110 health authority purchasing plans contained one or more contract exclusions; most of the procedures listed could be classed as marginal or ineffective services (cited in Mulligan 1998).

6 For example, cardiothoracic transplantation, craniofacial surgery services and extra corporeal membrane oxygenation. The NSCAG 'aims to help patients by improving access to uncommon services, whilst at the same time seeking to sustain high levels of expertise by preventing proliferation to too many centres. It aims to help local commissioners by smoothing out risk, and removing from them the responsibility to plan for the unplannable. And it aims to help providers by assuring a cash flow to support rare and expensive treatments, and by providing a focus for discussion about service development' (www.doh.gov.uk/nscag).

7 Proposals for establishing NICE in the UK were first set out in the white paper *The New NHS: Modern, Dependable* (Department of Health 1997) and further elaborated in the consultation paper *A First Class Service: Quality in the New NHS* (Department of Health 1998).

8 At the time of writing, research into the impact of NICE guidelines on clinical and managerial practice was due to be published in 2003. An assessment of the impact of one set of NICE guidelines (for surgical repair of inguinal hernias) found that the guidelines had had no impact on NHS practice (Bloor *et al.* 2003).

9 The rapid assessment of Relenza highlights a concern that while such an approach is said not to be a substitute for the formal appraisal process,

the effect of the recommendations of NICE will be just as significant. One commentator suggests that rapid assessments raise the 'potential for concertinaed time-lines resulting in an assessment that falls short of the declared aim of achieving a transparent and well-structured process' (Dodds-Smith 2000). To date only one rapid assessment has been undertaken.

10 The chief executive of NICE stated that, despite the use of numbered copies of appraisals and asking those consulted to sign legal confidentiality agreements, it had not proved possible to maintain confidentiality.

11 The guidelines for drug treatments (Viagra) for impotence were issued prior to NICE's existence, as described earlier.

12 Albeit with secondary considerations of the significant potential annual cost implications of the drug in England and Wales, which ranged from £7.6 million to £15.0 million (www.nice.org.uk/article.asp?a=427 (accessed 8 October 2002)).

13 Agenda and papers for the NICE annual public meeting, 18 July 2001.

14 The grounds for the appeal were that the guidance had overemphasized a single end-point (overall survival) in assessing clinical effectiveness in advanced breast cancer, applied unequal assessment of study data, and failed to provide adequate reasoning.

15 On the grounds that the statement in the *Guidance* relating to paclitaxel having 'no advantage in overall survival' was perverse because one specific study that was assessed was not designed to examine survival. The appellant also further argued that the *Guidance* was incorrect in inferring that mithromycin C was an anthracycline. Finally, the appellant claimed that the statement in the *Guidance* that paclitaxel showed 'no statistically significant advantage in terms of progression free survival after making adjustments for drug-related toxicity' was also incorrect and that the *Guidance* failed to recognize that paclitaxel and docetaxol are not the same.

6

NORWAY
Ole Frithjof Norheim

INTRODUCTION

Priority setting has been widely discussed within the health care system of Norway, at least since the mid-1980s. Two trends have followed in parallel: one of 'high-level activity' involving national commissions and white papers; and another with scattered attempts at priority setting at the micro and meso levels. Beside this, fair amounts of academic work on resource allocation have been published.

This chapter starts with a description of some attempts at setting priorities in Norway. It then examines experiences from Norway according to the seven questions set out in Chapter 1 of this book.

PRIORITY SETTING IN THE NORWEGIAN HEALTH CARE SYSTEM

Health care systems are fairly similar in the Nordic countries. The exact details vary, but in all countries the systems have almost exclusively been publicly funded through taxation, and most hospitals are also publicly owned and managed. In Norway, financing of hospitals is mainly the responsibility of the regional health authorities, although some hospitals and other institutions are owned and financed by the state (Nylenna 1995; European Observatory on Health Care Systems 2000).

Financing has traditionally been controlled through global budgets that are broken down into hospital budgets and then further divided among various hospital departments. Since 1997 a percentage of the expenses have been reimbursed according to the number and kind of patients treated. Norway has a fairly strong primary care sector (even though it varies in quality between the counties) where family physicians to various degrees act as gatekeepers to specialist services.

All insured persons are granted free accommodation and treatment, including medicines, in hospitals. This follows from the provisions of the Hospitals Act and the Act on Mental Health Care. In the case of treatment given outside hospitals, the provisions of the Act on Municipal Health Care and the National Insurance Act apply. The patient has to pay a share of the cost of treatment by a general practitioner or a specialist outside hospital, for treatment by a psychologist, for prescriptions of important drugs and for transportation expenses in connection with examination or treatment. The municipality and/or the National Insurance Administration cover the main part of the expenses. The patient's contribution (e.g. for an adult in connection with treatment by a general practitioner) is approximately £8 for each consultation, and 36 per cent of the cost of important drugs (maximum approximately £26 per prescription).

There are certain exemptions from the cost-sharing provisions for special diseases and groups of people. A ceiling for cost sharing is fixed by Parliament for one year at a time (about £115 in 2002). After the ceiling has been reached, a card is issued giving entitlement to free treatment and benefits for the rest of the calendar year.

The Lønning I Commission

In 1987 Norway was the first western country to develop national guidelines for priority setting in health care (Norges Offentlige Utredninger 1987). The committee responsible, led by Inge Lønning, was asked to consider five possible principles: the severity of the disease; equal access to treatment; waiting time; cost; and the patient's responsibility for their own health problem. It recommended that severity of disease should be the most important criterion for determining priorities, and it identified five separate priority levels (see Box 6.1). The report suggested that services in the two lowest priority groups should not be publicly funded before a satisfactory level of provision was achieved for the three highest groups. The details of this report are described elsewhere (Norheim 1995; Rolstad 1997; Ham and Locock 1998).

The emphasis on concerns for the worst off (the most severely ill)

Box 6.1   Lønning I Commission

First priority is given to measures which are necessary in the sense that there are immediate life-threatening consequences – for individual patients, patients groups or society as a whole – if the measures are not implemented immediately. Examples: emergency medicine (in surgery, internal medicine, and psychiatry), neonatal care.

Second priority is given to measures which are necessary in the sense that failure to carry them out will imply catastrophic or very serious consequences in the long run – for individual patients, patient groups or society as a whole. Examples: diagnosis and treatment of patients with severe and chronic diseases such as cancer, heart failure, severe rheumatic and orthopaedic diseases, care for the elderly.

Third priority is assigned to measures with documented effect, where the consequences of failure are obviously undesirable, but not as serious as those given first or second priority. Examples: patients with moderate acute and chronic health problems such as moderate hypertension; screening of groups with moderate risk factors.

Fourth priority is assigned to measures which are in demand, and are assumed to have health and life quality furthering effects, but where the consequences of not carrying them out are clearly less serious than is the case for measures of higher priority. Examples: high-technology medicine with poorly documented effect such as repeated ultrasound during pregnancy; medical treatment of common cold.

Zero priority is given to health services which are in demand, but are not necessary and do not have documented effect. Examples: high-technology medicine without known effect; screening of groups with no risk of disease.

---

is probably the report's main characteristic. Its guiding principle was expressed almost in Rawlsian terms: 'changes that improve the health status for the better-off groups should involve at least the same degree of improvement to the worse-off groups' (Norges Offentlige Utredninger 1987: 57). The Commission in particular emphasized the need to improve psychiatric services, habilitation and rehabilitation, long-term care and care for people with chronic illness.

Waiting-list guarantee

The most visible consequence of the Norwegian guidelines was the so-called waiting-list guarantee (passed by the Norwegian parliament in 1990). A guaranteed maximum waiting time of six months (reduced to three months in 1997) was based on the definition of priority group two (see Box 6.1): non-acute conditions for which delayed treatment would have catastrophic or severe consequences. The system has been evaluated in several studies (Skouen *et al.* 1989; Bjørndal and Guldvog 1996; Åbyholm *et al.* 1997; Kristoffersen and Piene 1997a, 1997b; Piene *et al.* 1997; Rasmussen *et al.* 1997; Piene 1998; Petersen *et al.* 1999). The high number of violations of the guarantee has been of constant political concern. Many clinicians have been against the regulations. Kristoffersen and Piene (1997a, 1997b), for instance, found that doctors interpret severity in different ways and that they are willing to reinterpret their patient's disease state if it will improve the patient's priority.

In a postal survey of 152 physicians and nurses in charge of allocating patients to waiting lists, Lian and Kristiansen (1998: 3921) found that the regulations imposed by the guarantee 'limit physicians' scope for setting priorities according to traditional criteria such as disease severity and admittance on a 'first come, first served basis'. They also argued (1998: 3926) that the results 'indicate that most respondents do not think that the reform has led to more equitable priorities. Health professionals seem to follow professional norms more than externally imposed rules'. Others (especially politicians) have pointed out that the existence of information on waiting time has directed attention to the health care system, thereby increasing pressure for reform (Norges Offenlige Utredninger 1997a).

Expert group developing national guidelines for bone marrow transplantation

Other health policy initiatives worked towards implementing the recommendations of the Lønning I Commission. At the clinical level, emerging high cost therapies led to the development of guidelines for bone marrow transplantation by an expert group appointed by the Health Council in 1990. The guidelines, published in 1992, explicitly built upon the Lønning I Commission and provided explicit criteria for selection of patients for transplantation (Helsedirektoratet 1992). The document also clarified which kinds of treatment options were given priority and which were considered experimental. At that time, the latter group included autologous bone marrow transplantation for all indications, including breast cancer and multiple myeloma, as well as allogeneic transplants with unrelated donors for patients with leukaemia above a certain age limit. The Health Council's mandate to the expert group included: to consider all applications from candidates for a bone marrow transplant; and to consider and adjudicate on appeals from patients denied this treatment and seeking coverage for treatment abroad. After this the patient could only appeal to the Ministry of Health. The expert group later asked to be relieved of the task of also considering appeals (Brinch *et al.* 1993).

Another expert group for high-dose chemotherapy with autologous bone marrow transplantation (later called stem cell support) was appointed in 1993. Its guidelines were published and implemented in 1995 (Statens Helsetilsyn 1995).

The Sandberg case

The explicit limiting of access to bone marrow transplants aroused public interest. The clinicians involved in the development of the guideline also applied it. The newspapers reported several cases of people who were denied costly high-dose chemotherapy followed by allogeneic (1992) or autologous bone marrow transplants (1994–95). Denial was justified with reference to the guideline and the reasons given there: incomplete evidence, high risks, small expected benefits and high costs.

The so-called Sandberg case was widely discussed in the media, and involved a medical doctor, then aged 53, who in 1992 was diagnosed with chronic myelogenous leukaemia (Karlsen 1993). His only chance of survival was allogeneic bone marrow transplantation with an unrelated donor. With reference to the national guidelines (developed, but not published at that time), and to international guidelines, he was denied a transplant as he fell outside the established indications (Executive Committee of the World Marrow Donor Association 1992). With an age limit around 50 years, treatment for this patient was considered experimental and too risky compared to the expected value of the outcome. Moreover, the expert group did not recommend that his expenses for treatment abroad should be covered. Following a massive media storm, the Minister of Health reversed this decision in 1993, and the patient received his treatment in Seattle, USA. He died a few months later.

The expert group defended their decision in several articles in newspapers and medical journals (Brinch *et al.* 1993). Reidar Lie, a professor of medical ethics, challenged both the decision and the ethical principles underlying the guidelines published in 1993. He argued they were based on utilitarian cost-effectiveness reasoning that could not expect support from all (Lie 1994).

It is interesting to note that after several cases of explicit coverage exclusions during that period, funding and the number of transplants performed increased significantly from about four transplants per 1 million inhabitants in 1992 to about eight in 1994 (Norheim 2000).

Publication of national guidelines for anti-hypertensive treatment

Guidelines with treatment recommendations with explicit cut-off values for anti-hypertensive treatment were also published in 1993 (Holmen 1993), and revised and expanded in 2000 (Meland *et al.* 2000). Although the consequences for public spending would be affected far more by these guidelines, compared to those for transplantation, there was little public interest in these issues.

National budget for investigational and experimental treatment

Norway implemented a programme in 1997, with ordinary public funding (outside the budgets of the Research Council), of large-scale clinical investigation of treatment effect and safety for new and 'promising' treatment modalities (Health Mo 1997).

The Matheson case

Another case that aroused interest from the public was that of a Norwegian woman with breast cancer with metastasis who in 1995 was denied high-dose chemotherapy with autologous stem cell transplantation in Norway because the treatment was considered experimental. She had this treatment in Sweden, but the National Insurance Administration refused to reimburse her costs. In 1996 the Minister of Health considered the matter and accepted her appeal, despite recommendations in national clinical guidelines as well as advice from oncologists and transplantation experts in the field (Nylenna *et al.* 1996).

One central issue in this debate was the problem of equal treatment for equal needs. The Minister of Health accepted the appeal from this woman partly because of delayed treatment of her appeal and partly because of new evidence published after the first treatment decision was taken (Bezwoda *et al.* 1995). He did not endorse a general policy of financing this treatment modality for similar cases.

The oncologists, on the other hand, argued that if she had treatment, all other patients in the same situation with similar expected benefits ought to have access to this treatment (Borud 1996a, 1996b, 1996c; Hernes 1996; Holte *et al.* 1996; Kolstad *et al.* 1996; Matheson 1996; Somdalen 1996). The expert group responsible for selecting patients according to the guidelines stopped work after its guidance was over-ruled, but accepted its responsibility again after some months.

Controversies encompassing new prescription drugs

Drugs considered 'important' are reimbursed, minus a user charge, by the National Insurance Administration. This is regulated by an annually published list which has two components. The first part lists conditions for which some drugs are considered necessary, and the second part lists the drugs (with some specification of the indications). The system for evaluation and review of new drugs is currently undergoing substantial changes. A main actor is the Norwegian Medicines Control Authority (SLK) which considers the effectiveness and safety of the drug in question. Decisions regarding reimbursement are taken in a separate process. Two new drugs, well known to international debate, have recently been added to the list of prescription drugs.

Donepezil for Alzheimer's disease

In 1998, the SLK approved the marketing of the drug donepezil (Stavrum 1998). The drug is said to improve mental capacities for patients with mild and moderate Alzheimer's disease for a period of time (about six months). Concern has been expressed about the quality of evidence, the magnitude and value of the outcome, and the costs of long-term use (Greenhalgh 1997; Kelly *et al.* 1997; Collier 1998; Melzer 1998). The Minister did not endorse its inclusion on the list of necessary drugs, but in 1999 Parliament approved the reimbursement from the year 2000 of 66 per cent of the costs (about £75 per year).

Alendronate as prevention against osteoporotic fractures

Alendronate was included on the list of prescription drugs in 1997, after much controversy between the different institutions responsible for decisions regarding uptake of new prescription drugs (Skogstrøm 1997). The benefits gained from this drug were considered marginal, compared to its costs, and the Ministry did not recommend its inclusion. A broad coalition within Parliament rejected the advice of the Minister of Health. One of the reasons given was that the majority in Parliament wanted to give higher priority to the group of patients (elderly women) typically affected by osteoporosis.

Interestingly, the SLK published an economic evaluation of the drug in its newsletter, reviewing the evidence on outcomes and costs. The pharmaceutical company marketing the drug in Norway (MSD) wanted the article withdrawn, arguing that it was misleading and based on unsound economic methods (Stavrum 1997). The company took the case to court, with the consequence that the article was withdrawn for a period, but the court eventually ruled in favour of the SLK.

The process of approval for these drugs has revealed the need to improve on the system, as has been argued in the latest White Paper on drug policies (Norges Offenlige Utredninger 1997b). As before, the National Insurance Administration (RTV) will be the authority that grants reimbursements for drugs. An evaluation of pharmacoeconomic consequences forms part of the consideration of applications for reimbursement. Pharmacoeconomic analyses were previously not a requirement in connection with applications for reimbursement, but have been so from January 2002. A transitional period was introduced up to this date with voluntary submission of analyses (Norwegian Medicines Agency 1999).

The Lønning II Commission

In 1996 a new commission was asked to revise the national guidelines of 1987. This second commission, also chaired by Professor Inge Lønning, had as its stated goal to recommend changes that could involve clinicians' day-to-day experience with limit-setting decisions. The Lønning II Commission recommends that changes to the current system of prioritization should take place from the bottom up. It proposes that specialty-specific working groups are established to make recommendations regarding priority setting within their own specialist fields and in accordance with predefined criteria of four priority groups: core services, supplementary services, low priority services, and services which should not be financed or reimbursed by the public health care system. (The definition of priority group I, core services, is given in Table 6.1.) A fifth priority group of 'investigative treatment' was also suggested for interventions that show promise, but where documentation is inconclusive and so funding should be considered separately.

Table 6.1   Definition of core services (Lønning II Commission)

Conditions A, B and C must be met.

A Health state (at least one of the following conditions must be met):

1. Loss of prognosis: The risk of dying from the disease within five years is greater than 5–10 per cent.
2. Diminished physical or mental functioning (or a significant risk of such a reduction): Permanent* and significant reduction in the patient's ability to perform tasks which he/she would generally perform in everyday life (occupational activity, schooling, housework, etc.), or tasks which patients in the same age group would normally perform.
3. Crippling pain that cannot be reduced sufficiently with the aid of non-prescription painkillers. One indication of strong pain is the diminished ability to carry out work and perform ordinary everyday activities (dressing, hygiene, sleep, cooking, etc.).

* The term 'permanent' means that the patient's state of health is not expected to improve without treatment.

B Expected benefit (at least one of the following conditions must be met):

1. Increase in the probability of five years' survival is greater than 10 per cent (absolute risk reduction).
2. Improved physical or mental functioning: Complete or partial restoration of previous state of health.
3. Reduction of pain which leads to improved level of functioning.
4. Nursing and care that can secure adequate nutritional intake, natural functioning, hygiene, dressing and the opportunity for external stimulus or social contacts.

C Cost-efficiency:

Costs should stand in a reasonable relation to the benefits of the treatment/care.

The working groups form part of a three-step process:

1. recommendations from working groups;
2. resource allocation by political and administrative decision makers;
3. formulation of clinical guidelines.

The guiding principles for all parts of the process are:

1. the severity of the condition;
2. the magnitude of expected outcomes from the intervention;

3. reasonable cost-effectiveness;
4. the quality of evidence on a scale of 1–3.

The Commission recommended that more emphasis should be placed on the second and third principles, as compared to the Lønning I Commission's emphasis on severity of disease.

The aim of these recommendations was to improve interaction between the political and clinical levels of decision making through processes that start at the bottom and go upwards – before returning to health personnel with day-to-day responsibility for using these guidelines. The Commission argued that the reliance on procedures at several levels of the decision making system is important 'because principles and criteria do not in themselves provide solutions to difficult rationing decisions. There is disagreement on the interpretation of evidence, and there are uncertainties and disagreement over which principles and criteria apply' (Norges Offentlige Utredninger 1997a: Section 8.1). The expressed idea is that 'a combination of guiding principles, fair procedures and appropriate medical judgements can secure the necessary legitimacy of the decisions made' (ibid.).

By 2002, few of the recommendations had been implemented, although a White Paper called 'Values for the Norwegian Health Services' recommended that the suggested procedures for priority setting should be implemented, and a standing commission for priority setting has been established (Sosial- og Helsedepartementet 1999b). The Minister of Health, in a newspaper article, also underlined the importance of establishing 'mechanisms for priority setting that can secure public support and legitimacy for the decisions that have to be made' (Høybråten 2000).

Adjustment of criteria for waiting-list guarantee

In 1997 there was an adjustment of the criteria for admittance to the waiting-list guarantee – partly based on the recommendations of the Lønning II Commission. The basic idea of these recommendations was informed by, among other things, the writings of Daniels and Sabin (Holm 2000). The Commission proposed a definition with criteria for deciding what kind of condition–treatment pairs should be assigned a guarantee. It also recognized that the definition had to be interpreted and applied in different clinical settings. It therefore advised that the criteria could be specified and tailored to specific conditions through a process involving clinicians, patients' groups and the public.

The Ministry took up the main elements of the definition (Table 6.1), but no processes were initiated. Instead, the Minister appointed another *ad hoc* working group. This group argued that medical discretion is most important in the process of assigning rights to patients. It advised against the proposal of a wide process:

> The working group believes this will be a very problematic process that in many ways will lead attention away from the total medical judgement that in all circumstances must be applied in these decisions. Guidelines based on a process, as suggested, will be impractical.
>
> (Rasmussen *et al.* 1997: 2212)

Instead, the group refined the definition, leaving its interpretation to the responsible decision makers.

Consequently, the then Minister of Health introduced three measures, some of them taking full effect only in 1998 and 1999. First, the criteria for who should have a guarantee were made stricter, according to the suggestions made by the *ad hoc* working group (Table 6.2). The time limit was at the same time reduced from six to three months (Sosial- og Helsedepartementet 1997). Second, the system for collecting information on waiting times from local, county and regional hospitals was radically improved. Third, and perhaps most importantly, the system for reimbursement of hospital costs was changed. Instead of a system based mainly on fixed

Table 6.2   Criteria for assignment of waiting-time guarantee (treatment within three months)

---

1. The patient expects a significant loss of time or loss of quality of life if treatment is delayed, that is,
   - ☐ significantly reduced time to live;
   - ☐ significant pain or suffering most of the time; or
   - ☐ significant problems with vital functions, such as nutritional intake or natural functions.

2. There is good evidence that time to live or quality of life can be
   - ☐ significantly improved by medical treatment;
   - ☐ significantly deteriorated without treatment;
   - ☐ permanently deteriorated because treatment becomes obsolete by delay.

3. There is a reasonable relation between costs and expected outcome.

Source: Ministry of Health (1997).

budgets, a percentage of the expenses is now reimbursed according to the number and kind of patients treated (Sosial- og Helsedepartementet 1998a). Between the end of 1997 and the beginning of 2001, the number of patients whose treatment violated the waiting-time guarantee fell from approximately 25,000 to around 5000–6000. For patients without a guarantee, waiting times have increased somewhat.

Norwegian Centre for Health Technology Assessment

Modelled on similar agencies in other countries, the Norwegian Centre for Health Technology Assessment (Senter for medisinsk metodevurdering, or SMM) was established as late as 1997 (Søreide and Førde 1998). The Centre was initiated and is financed by the Ministry of Health, and is organized as a non-profit independent research organization. Its main task 'is to critically review the scientific basis for methods used in health care, and to evaluate their costs, risks and benefits. Both new and established technologies will be assessed' (SMM 1999a: 5). Outputs in the form of reports are disseminated to defined target groups, policy makers, health care providers and patients.

By 2001, approximately 20 reports had been completed. Reports of special relevance to coverage decisions are concerned with screening for prostate cancer, thrombolytic medication for treatment of stroke, and heart laser treatment. The report on screening for prostate cancer notes that '[t]here are reasons to believe that widespread screening is quite common in Norway'. But, based on available evidence, the report concludes that 'routine screening of asymptotic men for early diagnosis of prostate cancer is not recommended' (SMM 1999b: 7).

In a similar vein, the report on thrombolytic medication for treatment of stroke concludes that 'the benefit of thrombolytic treatment in the studies assessed is uncertain and that additionally, intercranial haemorrhaging can occur as a complication to this form of treatment' (SMM 1999c: 5). The report also explicitly considers the issue of resource scarcity: 'furthermore, the treatment implies an ethical dilemma in that an expensive treatment with an associated relatively high risk for a few patients must be balanced against a possibly better end result for another group of patients' (SMM 1999c: 6).

A new treatment modality for angina pectoris, adopted in some countries, is transmyocardial laser revascularization, so-called heart laser treatment (SMM 2000). It has been considered experimental, but in 1994 a private hospital in Norway (the Feiring Clinic) asked for permission to offer this treatment to its patients, possibly as part of a randomized controlled trial. After considering the documented effect and risks, the Ministry of Health proscribed the method in 1995, but after considerable pressure in 1997 permitted and partly funded a randomized study by the National Hospital and the private hospital in question. A preliminary report on transmyocardial laser revascularization published in 1999 concluded that:

> Treatment with heart laser does not save lives. On the contrary, mortality related directly to the procedure is significant (3–20 per cent). Mortality appears to be particularly high among patients with unstable angina or cardiac failure. Survival after one year has been shown to be approximately the same in treatment and control groups in randomised studies.
>
> (SMM 2000: 5)

Summing up, these reports are all negative in the sense that they argue that the documented effect does not outweigh the risks (or costs) associated with the new technology in question. The reports have the status of 'recommendations' to the Ministry of Health and politicians as well as to clinicians working in the relevant field. Follow-up has not yet been evaluated. Since the work of the Centre is at an early stage and the number of technology assessments is small, it is not possible to assess the impact of the reports on clinical practice. Moreover, it should be observed that the conclusions are based on medical reasoning alone, using the criteria of evidence based medicine and Cochrane reviews for the assessment of the quality of evidence. Patient preferences or public opinion on acceptability are not considered explicitly and formally.

The Norwegian governmental appeal board regarding medical treatment abroad

Following the Matheson case (examined above), in 1997 the Minister of Health abolished the functions of the Ministry's advisory board with regard to medical treatment abroad, replacing it in 1999 with an independent governmental appeal board. Part of the rationale seemed to be a wish to remove such hard cases from the hands of the Minister (and consequently away from the interest of the media).

The National Insurance Act allows funding for treatment abroad only when there is a lack of competence within Norway, the condition is severe, and treatment is recommended by a tertiary-level hospital. Funding is not considered for interventions considered as experimental, except in cases where the number of patients is so small that one cannot expect to have large-scale randomized clinical trials in Norway. The appeal board is, according to its mandate, a kind of administrative 'court' presided over by a judge and with four members including medical doctors, representatives from the health service administration and patient organizations, as well as a medical ethicist (Sosial- og Helsedepartementet 1999a).

The Ministry of Health cannot reverse the decisions made by the appeal board. The only recourse for the patient is to bring the case before a civil court. During its first three years, the appeal board considered 184 cases. Of these, 21 decisions (11 per cent) were reversed (Norheim *et al.* 2002). A precedence archive of typical or especially interesting cases has been set up, and such cases are published on the Internet.

'ACCOUNTABILITY FOR REASONABLENESS'

This list of cases and documents relevant to priority setting in Norway is not extensive, but demonstrates particularly the 'complexity of rationing and the extent of unfinished business' (Ham and Coulter 2000: 233). In what follows, the experiences reported from Norway are examined according to the seven questions set out in Chapter 1.

What procedures are used to determine whether health technologies should be funded?

As reported above, there are few procedures that are established specifically with the aim of determining coverage decisions. Diffusion of new technologies is the rule, with some exceptions. For highly specialized interventions, such as transplants carried out at the National Hospital, coverage decisions are made with reference to the annual budget, and the Ministry of Health is directly involved in drawing up the final budgets. For other specialized diagnostic equipment or interventions, coverage decisions are partly incorporated in decisions regarding their level of provision (primary, secondary or tertiary care). Decisions are made in the Ministry, and also take into account advice from the Health Council's board for highly specialized treatment. For technologies used at lower levels of specialization, coverage exclusions are made at the county level, involving negotiations over the annual budgets.

Assignment of a waiting-time guarantee is the responsibility of the senior physician or nurse in each hospital department. There are no rules for how this judgement is to be made, and there is no possibility of appeal. The referring physician and the patient receive a letter informing them about the decision. Reasons are not required for assignment to the waiting list, but are sometimes stated briefly with reference to the relevant criteria (Lian and Kristiansen 1998).

Although an appeals procedure is in place for decisions of this kind, the lack of procedures for making the original decision – the decision not to offer a cartilage transplant or the latest chemotherapy – is striking. There are good reasons to believe that only a small portion of patients are denied treatment appeal.

What is the role of the different institutions in these procedures?

There are few institutions where rationing is considered the main issue. In one sense, and despite much 'high-level' activity in Norwegian health politics, rationing is a non-existent health policy issue. Few institutions are set up with this explicit aim. Moreover, regulation is centralized; funding is decentralized in Norway. This makes it difficult to identify institutions where such decisions take place. Probably the most important 'institutions' are the administrative and political decision makers at the county and regional level responsible for funding and providing health care through the hospitals. There is little research available in Norway on how these decentralized procedures at the meso level affect coverage decisions.

The newly established SMM gives advice on new technologies; it does not make coverage decisions (or have such a strong position as, for example, NICE has in the UK). As reported above, its recommendations are mainly based on work commissioned from expert groups. Before the Centre was established, related activities were organized by the Norwegian Research Council (McGlynn *et al.* 1990; Norwegian Consensus Conference on Mammography 1991; Waldenström 1995).

Decisions regarding uptake of new prescription drugs involve several institutions, including the Ministry of Health, the National Insurance Administration, the Health Council, and the Norwegian Medicines Control Authority. As pointed out in a recent White Paper, the division of responsibility between these actors is unclear (Norges Offentlige Utredninger 1997c).

What kinds of evidence do these institutions expect, require or consider in making funding decisions?

In Norway, following discussions after the Sandberg and Matheson cases, the distinction between experimental or investigational treatment on the one hand, and 'established' treatment on the other hand, has become important. The distinction has proved hard to clarify, but a consensus is forming.

In the work of the SMM, the Institute of Public Health and the governmental appeal board, evidence from randomized clinical trials, systematic reviews and meta-analyses is considered the gold standard for good quality evidence. The evidence hierarchy developed within evidence based medicine is increasingly referred to within the work of these institutions. Evidence from cost-effectiveness studies is often cited, but only as additional information in cases where evidence is considered incomplete.

There have been few coverage exclusions where there is conclusive evidence for a small treatment effect, but where an unfavourable cost-effectiveness ratio has been cited as the main reason. One exception might be the attempt not to include alendronate as a prescription drug for patients with established osteoporosis. Drug regulation is, however, probably the area where evidence on cost-effectiveness is most likely to be considered in the near future (Norges Offentlige Utredninger 1997c).

What 'standard of proof' do the institutions expect to be demonstrated in agreeing funding?

Except for the distinction between experimental and established procedures, no governmental institutions have explicitly formulated 'standards of proof'. However, the National Cancer Plan formulates a minimum standard of proof before any intervention should be regarded as established (Norges Offentlige Utredninger 1997c). These standards are related to the intention of treatment, and outcomes from the intervention are measured relative to standard treatment:

1. Treatment aiming for cure: 5–10 per cent absolute improvement in long-term survival (usually measured as five-year survival).
2. Treatment aiming for extended time to live: median survival improved by at least 20 per cent or a minimum of three months.
3. Treatment aiming for prevention of symptoms related to cancer: no minimum standard is defined, because there is no consensus on the relevant clinical endpoints.

4. Treatment intended for relief of symptoms: more than 20 per
   cent of the patients must have improvement of subjective
   symptoms such as pain, nausea, heavy breathing or other
   complaints.

These standards have been stated in previous and subsequent
publications in oncology, indicating that there is some consensus on
these standards developing among opinion leaders in the cancer
field (Statens Helsetilsyn 1994; Norheim *et al.* 1998; Kreftforening
IffoDN 1999). This is significant, given the large number of new
drugs now being evaluated.

What appeals mechanisms are available for reviewing decisions?

The new Patient Rights Act of 1999 includes the right to a second
opinion with regard to diagnostic and therapeutic interventions
(Sosial- og Helsedepartementet 1998b). The Norwegian governmental appeal board concerned with medical treatment abroad is the
only mechanism for appeal directly related to coverage exclusions.

To what extent does experience in Norway meet the tests of accountability for reasonableness set out by Daniels and Sabin?

Daniels and Sabin propose four conditions that need to be met to
ensure accountability for reasonableness: the publicity condition, the
relevance condition, the appeals condition, and the enforcement
condition (Daniels and Sabin 1997, 1998).

Publicity

Experience from Norway shows that the publicity condition is met in
only a few cases. In the cases taken up by the media, the argument
was in each case related to incomplete evidence. Scarcity of resources
was quoted only as an additional reason, if mentioned at all.

In cases involving bone marrow (or stem cell) transplants, the
rationale was more fully explained in the guidelines. It remains, however, an open question whether these guidelines can be considered
publicly accessible. Clinical guidelines, including the Norwegian,
tend to be formulated in a language inaccessible to the general
public, and they are not widely disseminated.

In most of the 184 cases considered by the governmental appeal
board during its first three years, the original decision was made with

reference to the experimental nature of the interventions in question. But there is nowhere the public can turn to search, read, assess or challenge this judgement, because the original decisions are not made public.

Information on coverage for prescription drugs is available in written form in the list of drugs reimbursed. Historically, this list has developed gradually. In principle, drugs that are deemed 'necessary' and costly in the long run for the patient are included (Norges Offentlige Utredninger 1997b). A more detailed rationale for inclusion and exclusion is not provided.

For highly specialized interventions, such as liver, heart and lung transplants, there exist no updated written guidelines, although indications can be deduced indirectly from papers in medical journals.

Relevance

Many of the same observations apply for the relevance condition. The rationale for coverage decisions, if available (as they are in recent SMM reports), rests on evidence, formulated as medical reasons. In those cases where the Ministry of Health reversed coverage exclusions (the Sandberg and Matheson cases), critics argued that the reasons were obviously 'political' (i.e. avoiding blame), because they did not apply to other and comparable cases.

Economic reasons (unfavourable cost-effectiveness ratios) are seldom cited in specific coverage decisions, although they are frequently invoked in general arguments about resource allocation. Moreover, whether the underlying principle of utility or health maximization is something 'all fair-minded parties can agree are relevant' remains an open question. This avoidance of almost any other explicit reasons for rationing than 'quality of evidence' should be of particular interest for policy analysis. It might suggest that all other reasons for rationing are considered politically contentious. Despite all 'high-level' activities, the need to ration 'effective' care is not acknowledged. As noted, justifications for rationing often rely on principles (such as the principle of maximization) that not even all fair-minded parties agree on (Daniels 1994; Norheim 1996, 2000; Holm 1998; Sabin 1998; Nord *et al.* 1999).

Appeals

In Norway, the courts play no part in decisions regarding coverage exclusions. The appeals condition is met only in cases regarding reimbursement for treatments abroad. Most importantly, there are no appeals mechanisms in place for coverage decisions regarding services within the country.

At the meso level, including the development of clinical guidelines, there is a tradition of a hearings process in Norway. The guidelines for bone marrow transplantation developed by the Health Council were subjected to a hearings process involving health professionals, governmental institutions and patient organizations before they were implemented. In theory, at least, these guidelines could have been challenged and revised accordingly. The hearings process does not, however, count as a formal appeal. The hearings are regarded as input to be considered in the decision on the final guidelines (Statens Helsetilsyn 1998).

The intermediate status of SMM reports is interesting here. Because they are seen as recommendations, not policy documents, there is little opportunity for revising these conclusions in light of further arguments. They will, however, be revised when new evidence accumulates.

Enforcement

Again, only in those few cases of coverage exclusions within the clinical setting has there been some voluntary regulation of processes. One could argue that the recommendations of the Lønning II Commission would change the system of priority setting in Norway towards a fulfilment of the first three conditions. The Ministry of Health has not implemented any of these. The enforcement condition has therefore not been met.

CONCLUSION: BETTER INSTITUTIONS OR MORE INFORMATION?

The experience from Norway shows political and administrative reluctance to introduce procedures and institutions with a mandate to make explicit coverage decisions. Even technology assessment is playing a minor role. In this respect, Norway lags far behind developments in New Zealand, the Netherlands and the UK.

The scattered attempts at improving procedures within the clinical setting show that improvements are possible, but without backing from central authorities such initiatives remain rare. What is emerging, however, is an increasing awareness that it is at this level –

the meso and micro levels of clinical and political decision making – that mechanisms of rationing have an impact. Here the potential for improvement is substantial.

What, then, about the focus on evidence based medicine? Unsystematic collection of information on outcomes, risks and costs will have little political impact if it is not done for a specific purpose. If such information could be systematized for groups of patients, with the specific aim of identifying patients who could benefit most from interventions and excluding patients where expected benefits are small and the costs are too high, the impact on resource allocation would be considerable. In this sense, the approach taken in New Zealand, the Netherlands and the UK with work on clinical guidelines appears promising.

To succeed along these lines, more systematic data collection on outcomes, risks and costs is needed in Norway. The growing interest in systematic evaluation of evidence according to the principles of evidence based medicine and health technology assessment should therefore be welcomed. What is needed in addition is to design channels where this information is made available and understandable to administrative and political decision makers. Recommendations based on evidence need to be tested against the goals and perspectives of a national health policy, and against the constraints imposed by the available resources (Norheim 1999). Such channels do not exist in Norway. Funding and coverage decisions at the meso level are not made according to outcome-centred criteria, but rather in line with historical budgets, broad investment considerations and uninformed expectations from the public. In short, the institutions necessary to create bridges between health policy and 'clinical policies' (the norms and practices of clinicians) are not in place.

From this perspective, it is easy to agree with Singer and others who have argued that for priority setting, governments and their institutions need to go beyond evidence based medicine and cost-effectiveness analysis (Singer 1997). Reliance on 'technical solutions' based on scientific reasoning will remain inadequate if not placed within the context of political procedures and institutions designed for coverage decisions. The choice is not, therefore, between stronger institutions and more information. Political and legal initiatives are needed to enforce public regulation of the processes of rationing. Stronger institutions will then increase the demand for more and relevant information. The challenge will be to clarify the roles of such institutions, so that relevant information and evidence is tested against political and economic considerations. By making both political and clinical actors accountable for each other's decisions, the first step towards horizontal accountability could be made.

The next step in Norway involves incorporating the requirements of a broader notion of deliberative accountability. This broader vertical accountability would imply that both clinicians and health authorities should be seen as accountable to the population they serve. The tests of accountability for reasonableness should be seen as helpful guidance in specifying what kinds of reasons those responsible for rationing should give to those who are affected by it.

7

THE NETHERLANDS

Marc Berg and Tom van der Grinten[1]

INTRODUCTION

This chapter discusses priority setting in Dutch health care. It starts with some facts and figures on the Dutch health care system. A brief history of priority setting in the Netherlands is then given, in which the seven questions raised in Chapter 1 will be explored. In the discussion we will examine one of the main findings emerging from this overview: that there is no single approach to priority setting. We will explicate the different approaches and analyse their assumptions, problem solving potential and application. Finally, we will summarize the discussion and examine where we can go from here, both theoretically and practically (i.e. how the rationing issue should be addressed politically and institutionally). We will argue that the challenge should be to accept the process of priority setting as the political process that it inevitably is, to find optimal ways to institutionalize this process with and within the health care system, and to feed the process with meaningful information.

FACTS AND FIGURES ON DUTCH HEALTH CARE

Funding

The 15.8 million inhabitants of the Netherlands collectively spent €34 billion on health care in 2000, or 8.8 per cent of gross domestic product, which is provided by approximately 875,000 health care workers (520,000 full-time equivalents). The financing of Dutch health care consists of a complex of different public and private programmes. Over 79 per cent of the funding is public (compulsory sickness funds, social insurance programmes and general taxation), and nearly 21 per cent private (private insurance schemes and direct payments by consumers of health care). On the public side only a very small element (4.4 per cent) is tax-based. The rest (74.8 per cent) is based on insurance premiums. This means that, although government has taken a firm grip on the size of these premiums and what they offer (the basic package), this is still not 'government money'. In other words, the insurance system creates a distance between the government and health care financing. It is the (private not-for-profit) sickness fund that fulfils the role of an intermediary organization, between government on the one side and the service organizations and professionals on the other. Contrary to the situation in the UK and Sweden, for example, the Dutch government does not generally exert any direct financial influence on health care expenditure.

Provision of health care

Hospitals and medical specialists

At the end of 1997 there were some 143 general (acute) teaching and specialist hospitals in the Netherlands, varying from small ones with fewer than 100 beds to big institutions with more than 1100 beds, with a total bed capacity of approximately 59,200.

A large majority (90 per cent) of hospitals are private not-for-profit organizations (for-profit hospitals are not allowed). The remainder (10 per cent) are publicly owned, including the eight university hospitals. To realize public goals within the private setting, the hospitals have been placed under strong planning, budgeting and quality regimes by means of a Health Charges Act, a Hospital Act and a Quality Act.

The approximately 13,000 medical specialists in the Netherlands are nearly all hospital-based. Only some specialists (such as psychiatrists) are allowed to practice outside hospitals. The rest are obliged to do their clinical and outpatient work within the setting of a hospital. This obligation was introduced without formal subordination of the specialists to the hospital management. Approximately 90 per cent, organized in mutual group practices or partnerships, act as private entrepreneurs in the general hospitals. The remaining 10 per cent are salaried members of the hospital organization.

Here we run up against one of the features of the organization of Dutch hospital care: the peculiar combination of separation and integration. The way the hospital management and the medical specialists are bound up within one hospital organization reflects the strong reliance in the Netherlands on professional autonomy and the expected benefits of co-operation. The concrete situation is characterized by a complex negotiating process within each individual hospital organization between medical specialists and hospital management, which are not bound in a hierarchical relationship.

Primary health care and home care

The Netherlands has a well-developed although fragmented system of primary health care and home care. The 7000 (full-time equivalent) general practitioners (GPs) are the key actors in Dutch primary health care. They co-operate in a more or less organized way with the 125 independent home-care organizations, which have a capacity of 53,500 full-time equivalent staff.

Not unlike the medical specialists, most GPs (90 per cent) are self-employed, organized in mutual partnerships or group practices. The remaining 10 per cent are employed on a salaried basis in health care centres, which are mostly run by private foundations or associations. GPs receive a capitation payment for their sickness fund patients and a fee-for-service from their privately (or non-) insured patients. GPs fulfil a screening role in Dutch health care for specialist and hospital referrals, which is obligatory for those with social insurance. Despite the capitation payment, referral numbers are not excessive by international comparison.

Long-term care

The Netherlands has a long tradition of hospitalizing psychiatric patients, the mentally handicapped, the disabled and the needy elderly in long-term care institutions. All these facilities are seen as part of the health care system. Although a move has developed towards a more differentiated supply of intramural, halfway and ambulatory facilities and so called 'living–caring combinations', levels of provision outside the hospitals and other institutions are not yet sufficient to absorb the growing demand for long-term care. The heritage of the institutional services – especially the 56,000 long-term care beds in the 324 nursing homes and the 117,700 places in the 1400 homes for the elderly – and the money they consume are still a barrier to necessary modernization in these sectors. The irony of the situation is that growing waiting lists for these very provisions actually lead to pleas (by consumers, politicians and service organizations) for more long-term beds and personnel.

The health care policy-making system

The Dutch state has major constitutional responsibilities for the efficiency, accessibility and global quality of health care, but it is in practice not equipped to accomplish these responsibilities under its own strength. An important feature of the health care policy-making system is in fact the absence of a power centre for implementing major policies, such as reforming the health care system or vigorously setting (new) priorities in health care.

The aforementioned characteristics – the way in which care is financed (insurance-based) and delivered (by self-employed professionals and private service organizations) – have given rise to striking interdependencies in the administration of Dutch health care. These interdependencies took shape in the intensive participation of private organizations in public policy making in a myriad of statutory bodies and less formal policy networks. Through these institutions the national associations of health care providers (doctors, hospitals, home-care organizations, etc.), insurers (sickness funds, commercial insurance companies), trade unions and employers' organizations have been able to play a remarkable role in the public policy arena by taking responsibility for the formulation and implementation of public policy and, by doing so, to legitimize governing authority towards their rank-and-file members (van der Grinten 1996).

This role of private organizations in public policy making is embedded in the broader co-operative (corporatist) traditions of the Dutch welfare state, nowadays known as the 'polder model'. The polder model is characterized by consensus between government, employers and trade unions (Peet 2002) and is so called after the process that led to the reclamation of new land (the polders) from the sea.

A BRIEF HISTORY OF PRIORITY SETTING IN THE NETHERLANDS

The history of priority setting in the Netherlands as a deliberate type of policy starts in the early 1980s. Four types of strategy can be distinguished:

- the introduction of medical technology assessment (MTA);
- the assessment of the basic package in the social insurance scheme;
- the use of waiting lists as one of the mechanisms for rationing health care; and
- stimulating the appropriate use of health care.

Although there is some historical sequence between these instruments and strategies – MTA and deliberations about a basic package typified the early days – they became more and more intermingled during the 1990s. At present all four are seen, or at least are seriously proposed, to be used in some combination in the priority setting activities of the different stakeholders in Dutch health care.

Medical technology assessment

In the Netherlands, the term 'medical technology assessment' is usually used rather narrowly, implying mainly the economic evaluation of medical technology. Although there was and still is much discussion about the importance of broadening this concept to include social, legal and ethical issues, in this chapter we will use the term 'MTA' in this narrow sense.

In the Netherlands, economic evaluations were introduced in the early 1980s by the Health Insurance Council (Ziekenfondsraad)[2] as a response to high-technology, high-cost health interventions such as heart and liver transplantation (Oortwijn 2000). All major new technological innovations, the Council suggested, were to be subjected to cost-effectiveness analysis (CEA) before coverage in the benefit package could be considered. This notion, that MTA could be of vital help for government priority setting, was broadly underwritten by other advisory bodies, leading to the establishment of the Fund for Investigative Medicine (Fonds Ontwikkelingsgeneeskunde) in 1988 (Boer 1999; Oortwijn 2000). This fund, administered by the Health Insurance Council, is the main Dutch MTA programme (Elsinga and Rutten 1997). Its aim is to fund research that will generate the information required for evidence based policy making at the national level and evidence based use of health care technologies at the practice level (Elsinga and Rutten 1997). It obtains its resources (about €16 million per year) mainly from the Ministries of Health, Welfare and Sport, and Education, Culture and Science.

Although these resources are substantial, they are insufficient to investigate all new major health technologies. Priorities, then, have to be set here as well: which technologies should be subjected to MTA in order to maximize the potential benefits of MTA in terms of overall health care quality and costs? At first, the Fund focused on the new, sophisticated technologies that lay at the root of its inception, such as heart transplantation and *in vitro* fertilization (Mulder 2000). These priorities were not picked out in advance: rather, they were suggested by researchers submitting proposals. After several years, dissatisfaction with this 'bottom-up' generation of priorities led to an attempt to determine priorities in a more top-down manner.

For this purpose, the Health Insurance Council in 1993 involved some 30 experts in a two-round Delphi procedure, generating a list of 126 routinely used services (e.g. diagnosis of and therapy for herniated lumbar disc, long-term psychotherapy, treatment of leg ulcers and palliative treatment in oncology) where doubts existed about their cost-effectiveness (Mulder 2000). The technologies on this list were then ranked. Different advisory bodies (such as the Health Council (Gezondheidsraad) and the Advisory Council on Health Research (Raad voor Gezondheidszorgonderzoek) have generated rather different rankings over the past seven years, including several wholly new lists (Niessen *et al.* 2000; Oortwijn 2000).

In addition to the Fund, the Dutch Health Research and Development Council (ZON) and the Netherlands Organization for Scientific Research (NWO) also fund MTA research. These organizations generate topics for funding in a variety of ways, including direct input from the Ministry or input from expert working groups that formulate funding programmes. Overall, then, the identification and priority setting for MTA studies in the Netherlands is complicated and patchy (see Figure 7.1) and the use of its outcomes (like the rankings) in actual policy making is still modest (see below).

The impacts of the MTA studies are many and varied. MTA studies have contributed to government decisions to introduce, for instance, pancreas and lung transplantation and extra-corporeal membrane oxygenation. Yet these impacts have been far from

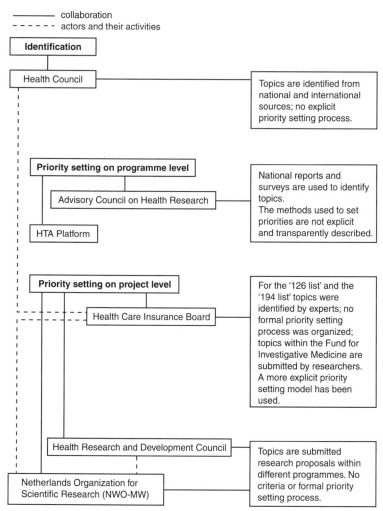

Figure 7.1   Relation between actors involved in identification and priority setting for health technology assessment in the Netherlands

(*Source*: Oortwijn 2000: 105)

unequivocal (van Rossum 1991; Elsinga and Rutten 1997). Although it is definitely the case that these studies have generated arguments used in political debates, and have created an overall awareness of the importance and relevance of economic arguments, there are not many examples of tough policy decisions that were decided by one or several MTA studies. Sometimes an MTA study will corroborate a decision already in the making; sometimes an MTA study will remain unused because, for example, the research question is too far removed from the policy question at stake.

Most often, however, technologies are introduced without any MTA evaluation. Sometimes, also, technologies that were proven to be not cost-effective were allowed anyway – as happened in the case of lung transplantation (Rutten 2000). In a recent example, the situation was exactly the opposite: whereas a high-quality MTA study had proven the cost-effectiveness of Viagra as a treatment for erectile dysfunction (the cost per QALY was in fact far less than in the case of many well-established health technologies), the Minister decided to exclude it from the basic package (Stolk *et al.* 2000a, 2000b). In this case, the expected total financial impact of the introduction of this new technology on the health care budget had more political weight than the outcome of the MTA analysis.

On the level of health care practice, the synthesis and distribution of MTA study outcomes are handled primarily by the health care professions (Mulder 2000) through the inclusion of MTA study results in guidelines. Whereas professional bodies have enthusiastically embraced the importance of including evidence of effectiveness in their guidelines, they are only now beginning to include economic considerations.[3]

Assessment of the basic package in the social insurance scheme[4]

In 1991 the Dutch Committee on Choices in Health Care produced what has since then become known as the Dunning Report, named after its chairman (Committee on Choices in Health Care 1992). Although all four instruments and strategies mentioned above were addressed in the Dunning Report, the main focus was on the assessment of the basic benefits covered in the social insurance package.

The report argued as follows. Scarcity in health care is inevitable. While inefficiencies certainly need to be combated, this will at best resolve the scarcity problem only temporarily. Expanding the available budget (or increasing social security premiums) may be required but is only possible to a limited extent because of competing claims on public revenues. The problem of priorities cannot therefore be evaded, at least as long as the principle of equal access to health care is maintained without rendering health care unaffordable. The Dunning Committee added a further question: must everything that is technically possible in health care in fact be offered and, if so, to what extent must all this be publicly funded? This question marked a fundamental shift from health care in a general sense to what might be termed 'necessary care'.

The Dunning Committee subsequently arrived at the following basic principles. First, it is fairer to ensure necessary health care for all than for just a proportion of the population to have access to all conceivable medical facilities. Second, an explicit and publicly accountable choice is better than covert rationing. Third, in setting priorities in health care, authentic social values must be combined with professional and expert opinion as to what is meaningful and meaningless medical treatment.

The report developed four criteria to apply in succession in order to remove obsolete existing types of care from the benefits package and prevent inappropriate new types of care from entering the system. Taken together, these criteria were called 'Dunning's funnel':

1. Is it necessary care (from a community point of view)?
2. Has it been demonstrated to be effective?
3. Has it been demonstrated to be efficient?
4. Can its payment be left to the responsibility of the individual?

This strategy for priority setting and the criteria to be used ran into severe criticism after the publication of the report. The most important points of criticism were as follows (van den Burg and ter Meiden 1998):

- The broad definition of health and the contested definition of 'necessary' made it difficult to pinpoint which facilities did and did not form part of necessary care and hence the basic package.
- Which facilities can and which cannot be left to the individual patient to pay for vary from case to case and cannot therefore be readily determined at the macro level.
- The utilitarian nature of Dunning's approach (i.e. the preference for services from which the largest possible number of members of society benefit) subordinates the individual to the community.
- Only a few services can be said to be entirely ineffective or inefficient; effectiveness and efficiency depend on the medical indication, which cannot be properly determined at the macro level.

What is striking about this criticism is that it relates in particular to the two politically most sensitive criteria: the individual affordability of health care and the determination (and thus limitation) of 'necessary' care. The criteria of effectiveness and efficiency were more warmly received, but the political and public noise surrounding the assessment of the basic package pushed this to the background. The former government of Christian Democrats and Social Democrats stated that although the contents and scope of the package of services should be a political decision, the Dunning Committee criteria were not usable for this purpose. It took measures to include all types of care that it considered essential in a basic package: approximately 95 per cent of the then present health care services.

When a new government coalition of Liberals, Social Liberals and Social Democrats took office in 1994 (this coalition served for the rest of the period under discussion), the previous government's plan for a basic package of 95 per cent was immediately pushed aside. This meant that Dunning's approach got a second chance. The latter did not, however, prove particularly successful. Apart from the problematic substantive criteria of the Dunning Committee, financial considerations (i.e. the need for spending cuts and the anticipated return of the measure in question) and political pressures (from political parties and interest groups) made it very difficult to remove services from the package.

Waiting lists as a mechanism of rationing health care

The government managed to keep the thorny question of waiting lists off the political agenda for several years after the publication of the Dunning Report. Although there were waiting lists, the fact that the waiting lists and waiting periods were not properly and uniformly recorded and that opinions as to their causes and consequences diverged meant that the scale of the problem could not be clearly determined. In the mid-1990s, however, two developments served to highlight the issue: services were offered on top of the compulsory package, open to private insurance or out-of-pocket payments; and priority access was given for services in the compulsory package to a specific, eligible population, with extra funding.

The first development was a form of privatization outside the mainstream provision (i.e. paid through social insurance or via earmarked payroll taxes), and applied especially to nursing and home care and private outpatient clinics. These offer facilities outside mainstream health care for those able and willing to pay for them out of their own resources or via private insurance. This development has become a highly controversial one. Nevertheless privatization is still continuing in this area, albeit in the shadow of mainstream health care. A system of private home nursing is arising which is used not just by the well-off but also, notably, by mainstream health care in order to ease the pressures on the system.

The second development was a form of privatization inside the social insurance package. A reform of the Dutch social insurance system in 1996 acted as the trigger, in that this reform placed the financial risk of long-term sickness absence on the employer. This gave employers a very real incentive to return their employees to good health. It then rapidly became clear that waiting lists cons-tituted an obstacle. This transfer gave employers a financial interest in effective and, in particular, swift delivery of health care. The incentive on the part of employers set in motion a stream of initiatives to bypass the waiting lists in mainstream health care. The most prominent of these have been specific outpatient clinics, where the employees of a particular firm can receive swift treatment in return for payment and so can return to work quickly.

These initiatives on the part of businesses and hospitals to get around the waiting-list problem sparked off a fundamental political and public debate, in which the preferential treatment of employees (ahead of those not in employment) was heavily criticized. Company outpatient departments, although still of negligible importance in practical terms, evolved into the leading symbol of the threatened bifurcation of Dutch health care into a private (read 'fast' and 'expensive') and a public (read 'slow' and 'underperforming') domain. Fundamental values of equity and solidarity were seen as being at issue. As had happened previously in the case of home care, the possible practical benefits were overruled by the threat of legislation banning hospitals from giving preferential treatment to employees. This has partly been realized by legalizing existing private clinics, which implied that these clinics are bound by the same rules as 'ordinary' services.

In 1998 the governing political parties and the health care organizations reached agreement on a plan of approach. This plan provided for a financial injection, a number of structural measures and agreement that employees were not to be given priority. Hospitals were to receive money to alleviate the worst bottlenecks, on condition that they submitted properly worked-out proposals and took structural measures to reduce waiting lists. If they failed to come up with results, the flow of money would be stopped. An additional €59 million a year has been set aside for these project subsidies, topped up by even more money in recent years. The structural measures, which are intended for the entire curative sector, consist of the uniform recording of waiting lists, clear-cut medical and urgency indicators, encouragement of co-operation between health care institutions, the rearrangement of care processes and longer working hours.

In sum, the process of handling the waiting lists is mainly left to the creativity and tenacity of the individual service providers – home care, nursing homes, hospitals and professionals. The social insurance companies are, at best, supporting the suppliers' initiatives and government remains preoccupied with the ideological debate on the impending division of society if private clinics and special treatment for employees are accepted. The growing pressure on government to do something did not result in it taking a firm lead in tackling the waiting lists. Instead government is still offering (lots of) extra money to the providers, connected with a mass of bureaucratic conditions on spending. These are evidently not the policy conditions that are needed for a process of accountability for reasonableness.

Appropriate use

At much the same time as the Dunning Committee issued its report in 1991 the Health Council issued a report concerning the effectiveness and efficiency of medical treatment (Health Council of the Netherlands 1991). This report was prepared under the leadership of the subsequent Minister of Health and then vice-chairman of the Health Council, Dr E. Borst. Since the effectiveness of health care is not so much concerned with treatments *per se* as with their application by doctors to patients, medical treatment occupied a central place in this report. The Health Council identified a lack of knowledge about the cost-effectiveness of diagnosis and therapy as the major obstacle in the effectiveness of health care. Many treatments whose usefulness has not been demonstrated are routinely performed. Insurers contribute to this as their payouts are based not on proven cost-effectiveness but on the criterion of established practice. On this basis the Health Council arrived at the recommendation to stimulate the creation and use of guidelines based on the results of cost-effectiveness research.

As Dr Borst became Minister Borst, this approach evolved into the main thrust of government policy concerning health care choices. Instead of setting priorities at the macro level of the system, the focus of policy shifted towards the meso and micro level, where the health service professionals, institutions and health care insurers were encouraged to promote the appropriate use of the scarce resources (Borst-Eilers 1998). The professional community had already broadly invested in peer review, pharmacotherapeutic consultations, education and training, consensus building and guidelines. The Minister in turn supported these efforts by encouraging MTA and the application of its results. As we go on to discuss, however, the number of guidelines explicitly incorporating cost-effectiveness information is still very low.

PRIORITY SETTING POLICIES: THE GLOBAL PICTURE

The way in which the Netherlands deals with the issue of choices in health care is through a gradual, incremental approach. It is a patchy assembly of diverse procedures, standards of proof and institutions, in which use is made of a mix of strategies and shared responsibilities, with an important role for the actors at the meso and micro levels.

MTA analyses are carried out to guide national policy, yet the list of excluded services is still minimal and highly eclectic. Echoing experiences in other countries, few services have been excluded from Dutch public health insurance coverage – no matter how thorough and formal the evaluation of the technology. The setting of national priorities appears to be a difficult process, in which political, economic and moral considerations become intertwined. Nevertheless, the rise of MTA and Dunning's funnel has been very significant. There is now widespread recognition that we have to 'develop acceptable ways of resolving the tension between increasing demands and limited public financial resources' (Mulder 2000: 329).

Yet, in line with developments in other Western countries, government health policy has recently shifted its focus to emphasizing clinical guidelines and evidence based medicine. Rather than limiting the basic health care package through a process of priority setting, the emphasis is now on attempting to influence the individual treatment decisions of clinicians through evidence based guidelines. As Mulder (2000: 329) puts it, 'rather than excluding services from public health insurance coverage, the emphasis is now on ensuring that the services included in the basic package are used appropriately'. Now that governments do not seem to be able to indicate what 'appropriate care' is, attention is turning to ensuring that the individual health care professional's activities are 'appropriate'. This has been labelled the 'turning over' of the funnel, since the focus has shifted from making choices between care options in the package at the national level to choices within categories of care options at the clinical level (Mulder 1997).

Taken together, however, the plethora of more or less formal approaches to priority setting – whether targeted at limiting the package or at optimizing its utilization – has not resulted in the disappearance of the scarcity problem that led to all these activities. As a pragmatic 'solution', the government has not abandoned the tried and trusted policy of national rationing (i.e. keeping the production capacity limited and setting a ceiling on production in order to resist the pressure on the public system of Dutch health care). Having waiting lists might not be a very rational way of prioritizing health technologies – it could nevertheless be a practical way of doing so, which might even at times meet the criteria of 'accountability for reasonableness' (Daniels and Sabin 1998).

ASSESSMENT OF STEERING MECHANISMS AND PROCESSES FROM A 'RATIONAL' PERSPECTIVE

Insufficient co-ordination

When looked at as a 'steering model' for the decision to use or acquire new medical technologies, the 'system' that is in place (if we can call it that) is very loose. First of all, there is no central direction by which technologies are targeted for MTA. There was the '126 list' of the Health Insurance Council, which is by itself just a list to which other organizations may or may not orientate themselves, and which has itself been prioritized and renewed in different ways (see Table 7.1). The Health Insurance Council's Investigative Medicine Fund, in fact, has been taken over by the Netherlands Organization for Scientific Research, but it is still flanked by the manifold research and implementation programmes of the Health Research and Development Council. In addition, there may be many other local and national initiatives, funded through different routes, that do MTA studies or set up trials generating information relevant for guideline construction.

The most important guideline development programmes are those of the Dutch Institute for Health Care Improvement (CBO) and the Dutch College of General Practitioners (NHG). These programmes encompass a broad range of topics (covering specialist care, GP care and, to a lesser extent, multi-disciplinary care) but do not themselves fund or carry out MTA research. Until very recently, there was little,

Table 7.1 Top five priorities indicated by different actors involved in identification and setting priorities for HTA

A. Priorities from the Health Council, derived from the '126 list', as described in the annual working programme for 1999
1. Incontinence
2. Chronic use of benzodiazepines
3. Decubitus
4. Use of devices in physiotherapy
5. Long-term psychotherapy

B. Priorities from the Advisory Council on Health Research and the Committee on Explorations, as published in a report on exploring priorities in health research in 1996
1. Diagnosis and treatment of chronically ill: e.g. mental problems in children and adolescents; adults and depression
2. Adequate care of diseases which occur in the elderly, impairments: endocrine aspects of ageing, dementia and CVA
3. Stimulating autonomy and self-care: the patient as actor in health care and home-care technology
4. Primary and secondary prevention: innovative prevention, effectiveness and efficiency of preventive technologies and implementation
5. Quality and efficiency of care: evaluation of medical practice, clinical decision making regarding diagnostics and quality of care

C. Priorities from the Advisory Council on Health Research as described in the advice on HTA, 1998
1. HTA research into the economic aspects of existing technologies (especially topics on the '126 list'), new technologies including medical aids, and drugs
2. HTA research which covers not only the efficacy (and possible costs) but also other aspects, such as regional and individual differences in the care provided, highly complex care, the national policy on quality of health care and the macro-economic impact of (new) health technologies and/or care technologies
3. HTA research into prevention and diagnostic procedures
4. HTA research into nursing and paramedical care facilities
5. HTA research into mental health care facilities

D. Priorities from the '126 list' as published by the Health Care Insurance Board in 1993
1. Ultrasound treatment for problems of the locomotor system
2. Treatment and cure of non-hospitalized acute psychiatric patients
3. Specialist care for chronic patients
4. Diagnosis of suspected hernia nucleus pulposa
5. Diagnostic arthroscopy of the knee compared to diagnostic magnetic resonance imaging (MRI)

Source: Oortwijn (2000: 103)

if any, formal co-ordination between these development programmes and MTA funding organizations. The need for more co-operation has been recognized, but the Dutch 'polder model' ensures that concrete changes in actual practices will be slow.

Furthermore, there are few guidelines for guidelines. That is to say: the Health Care Improvement Institute, the General Practitioners' College and other national or local guideline-producing agencies (regional cancer centres, local hospitals, specialist groups, para-professional groups – both locally and nationally) act in their own ways, and only recently have they started to discuss the need to co-ordinate activities with each other. There are CBO guidelines and NHG guidelines for the same conditions, for example; and only recently have efforts been undertaken to ensure that the two guidelines do not contradict each other. Also, there are so far very few CBO or NHG guidelines that formally incorporate MTA data.[5] All the other guidelines are based only on efficacy or effectiveness data, which implies that, from a policy perspective, these are highly limited tools when it comes to 'steering' the use or acquisition of (new) medical technology.

There is thus, little formal co-ordination between these guideline-producing bodies with respect to targeting, the content or form of the guidelines, or their dissemination or potential enforcement. Nor has there been much co-ordination with the agencies that set priorities for MTA and fund MTA research (who themselves are only poorly co-ordinated with each other – although a recently established 'MTA platform' should change this). Although the importance of the incorporation of MTA results in guidelines is widely recognized, and although large subsidies are given for the creation of evidence-based guidelines, there is as yet no structural financing of the MTA research that should be incorporated in these guidelines.

There is, in addition, no real enforcement of any of the produced guidelines. Outside of experimental situations, there are very few instances where a treatment will only be funded when a specific protocol is followed. All other guidelines so far are just that: 'guiding principles', to be used and interpreted at the doctor's discretion. Importantly, studies that investigate the impact of such guidelines on actual decision making lead one to be rather sceptical (Kosecoff *et al.* 1987; Klazinga 1994). Dutch GPs are often not even aware of the content of specific guidelines, let alone allowing their actions to be influenced by them. As a result, much work is now being done to study how to implement guidelines optimally (drawing upon techniques from social psychology, diffusion research and marketing studies), so that health care professionals will actually start using them (Grimshaw *et al.* 1995; Grol 1997; Health Council of the Netherlands 2000).

Missing the normative and values dimension

If cost considerations are rarely systematically incorporated in guidelines, other normative considerations (concerning, for example, issues of justice, solidarity, the patient's voice in the decision making process and so forth) are even less well represented. This comes back to the debate on the 'narrow' definition of MTA that is prevalent in priority debates. Most guidelines may indicate whether an intervention is 'evidence based' – yet they would rarely state whether and when the intervention would be 'necessary' from a broader normative or value perspective (such as the position of Dunning's 'collective'). An intervention aimed at preventing disease in low-risk individuals may be 'evidence based', but this does not answer the question whether this intervention is 'appropriate'. Screening for diabetes might be effective, but such a conclusion leaves unresolved whether this would be a wise way to spend scarce resources. An evidence based guideline, in short, is not in and of itself 'value-based', and formulating guidelines for 'effective care' is not a solution to society's problem of 'appropriate care' (Berg *et al.* 2001).

Health care technology decision making as a political process

All in all, then, this is very 'indirect' steering indeed. It is a far cry from a rationalist, explicit approach to health care technology decision making, in which the ideal situation would be one in which quality-adjusted life years (QALYs) could be calculated for every possible intervention for any given condition. This is the ideal that often underlies calls for more information, for more generalizable technology assessments, for more rational priority setting: to work towards a fully rational policy in which every euro spent on health care interventions buys an approximately equal and optimal amount of QALYs.

Yet, we argue in accord with a growing number of other authors, priority setting is necessarily messy and difficult. It is inescapably a political process, that is to say, a decision making process which takes into account issues of interest and values, taking place under conditions of urgency and uncertainty. There are several reasons for this conclusion; many of which are dealt with extensively elsewhere (Klein 1992, 1998; Hunter 1993, 1995, 1997; Harrison and Hunter 1994; Mechanic 1995; Klein *et al.* 1996; Ham 1997; Daniels and Sabin 1998; Day and Klein 1998; Ham and Locock 1998; Holm 1998; Coulter and Ham 2000). We have already pointed at a few fundamental observations.

First of all, doing a cost-effectiveness analysis (CEA) or making guidelines involves making all kinds of normatively charged assumptions and translations. Rather than undoing the need to make political prioritizing or rationing decisions, the process of CEA and guideline production can make these choices more visible (in the best case) or hide them from view and bury these choices in the seemingly 'rational' CEA and guideline (in the worst case). CEAs are only about 'costs', moreover, leaving all the other normative considerations that go into setting optimal criteria for diagnosis and treatment to be dealt with 'implicitly' in the guideline-construction or priority setting process.[6]

The fundamental problem here is that health care does not have one 'goal': it contains a 'complex composite of many goals, including fuzzy goals such as maintaining a sense of security in the population' (Holm 1998: 1001). Other 'goals' can be more individual, such as reassurance, improvement of quality of life, the need for a last hope, and so forth. These goals are variable and context-dependent, making their explication and formalization over and above individual situations excruciatingly difficult. Most important, however, is that it would be an illusion to think that these goals could be ranked or grouped in any harmonious way. Not only are they fluid – depending on the individual, on the situation – they are also in perpetual tension with one another; always competing for priority.

On a more mundane note, it would be just impossible to do (and keep up to date) all the CEAs and produce the evidence based guidelines that we would like to see. This problem is enormous. It will not even be possible to focus comprehensively on even a few of the most costly and problematic issues of the '126 list', unless a few crucial decision points are selected. The information ('evidence') is simply lacking; the calculations for comprehensive CEAs simply become too complex (van Hout *et al.* 1999). Put in economic terms, the cost of doing so would outweigh the potential benefits.

Blame shifting

The rather technocratic idea that we can rationally establish appropriate care and decide on scarcity issues has a problematic edge to it when we look at the move from setting priorities at the national level to achieving 'appropriateness' through guidelines for practitioners. This 'pushing off' of political responsibility is legitimated by pointing at the 'technical solution' that CEAs and guidelines promise (at least in the eyes of many policy makers – most CEA analysts and guideline writers are not so naive). Yet, as we argued above, these instruments do not solve these issues – they bring them into the open, or displace them from one decision context to another.

One important danger of this development, then, is that the whole array of normative/political considerations linked to the question whether a treatment should or should not be available may be pushed down from the macro to the meso or micro level (Mulder 2000). Rather than being technically 'solved', hard decisions about whether or not to spend resources on treating individual patients, or the weighing of contrary normative considerations (such as equity and utility) will end up in the doctor's office. At the very least, at the macro level, in priority setting debates and attempts, political and ethical considerations are discussed openly.

Often, of course, these issues are so conflict-prone that no solution can be found; indeed, the plurality of values and the politically charged nature of rationing decisions are often mentioned as the prime reasons for the failure of priority setting attempts. Yet what happens when priority setting is more or less abandoned, and attention focuses on ameliorating decisions of individual doctors? Rationing decisions will of course still be made, but now implicitly, by individual physicians, or behind closed doors by hospital boards (e.g. in the case of budget shortages). Put critically, abandoning priority setting attempts at the macro level shifts the burden of responsibility to individual physicians and institutions.

Without any further conditions this could be highly problematic because such decisions are thereby made outside of any sphere of public accountability and democratic control. In addition, those having to make these decisions are put in a position which is highly undesirable, both from their own perspective and from a more policy-oriented perspective. They have to make rationing decisions while faced with the needs of individual patients, without having recourse to publicly underwritten criteria. This leads to an impossible 'double bind' for the health care professional, and to inequality in decisions made – an inequality which remains invisible since all these decisions remain implicit.

Policy talk and practice[7]

Examining the way in which Dutch health care policy is conducted and decisions are reached brings us to a significant paradox in Dutch government policy in recent years with respect to the choices in health care. The rhetoric and deployment of this policy are permeated with the need to be as rational and explicit as possible in decision making concerning medical treatment at the various levels. Evidence based medicine and explicit knowledge – these are what is at issue. But this strict approach is applied in a practical situation that is heavily dependent on professional involvement at the lowest level of care, on the barely enforceable co-operation of institutions and care insurers at the meso level and on a consensus-building type of policy making at the macro level.

In this respect we should repeat that the government's position in Dutch health care is not a powerful one. Instead there are marked mutual dependencies in the system between government, the private (not-for-profit) service organizations, independent professionals and private insurers. This is why trust, consensus and co-operation are such important policy instruments in Dutch health care. Although the positions in this system are changing – the traditional social orientation of the private sectors (service organizations, insurers) is shifting towards a more strategic and sometimes commercial one, while new stakeholders (e.g. employers' organizations) are entering the field without the legacy of strong feelings for the traditional values in health care – these strong dependencies and the associated policy practices still characterize most of the decision making processes in Dutch health care.

What is striking is that the formal policy hardly takes into account these potentialities, and the implicit or tacit knowledge within this system, especially at the meso and micro level. That is to say, the repertoire of personal skills of those concerned in health care and their experience, imagination and intuition are barely drawn on. On the contrary, there is a preoccupation with erasing these 'subjective' factors so that it becomes possible to manage on the basis of explicit knowledge laid down in rules, procedures, protocols and manuals. As Weggeman (1997: 20–1) argues:

the lamentable thing about this preoccupation is that it necessarily results in addiction, for as long as we are dealing with people, the process of objectification will never be completed, even in the tiniest field of endeavour. This kind of work takes a great deal of time . . . and holds back renewal and innovation.

DISCUSSION

We cannot rest contented with the conclusion that the 'informal' decision procedures established in Dutch health care will prevail, that they will withstand the strong rhetoric about rationality and formal decision procedures, and will thus keep everything working. That would be unfounded romanticism: we have pointed to the current government's problematic tendency to delegate priority decisions to individual professionals and institutions, and we have indicated that this was partly legitimated by the government's belief in its own formal discourse. What do we need in order to make decisions on health care technologies, if not more explicit information and more formal decision models?

We would argue that you cannot rationally make 'choices' a starting point of your policy (i.e. following the MTA book as the policy makers like to read it). A fully 'rational' approach is not possible at the macro level, nor at the meso or micro level. You have to institutionalize the existence of the pluriformity of values and the crucial uncertainty that will always thwart any such attempt (rather than attempting to erase this pluriformity and undo this uncertainty). You have to be creative and eager in exploiting the given possibilities in the policy-making institutions in Dutch health care, drawing upon the 'polder' traditions.

There are no simple answers when it comes to a 'choice' for or against a new medical technology – and you will have to design your policy starting from this insight, rather than seeing this situation as a temporary nuisance that will be overcome by sufficient funding resulting in 'better information'. We will conclude by pointing to the routes such an approach could take. Before doing so, however, we will first address the question of to what extent the experiences in the Netherlands meet the test of 'accountability for reasonableness', as set out by Daniels and Sabin (1998).

Publicity

Two mechanisms seem relevant in this respect: publicity and public involvement. Although there is considerable and growing attention in the mass media in medical affairs – in this respect the Netherlands is no different from other countries – information about rationing decisions and their rationales is barely available. The reasons are obvious since, in a situation without clear-cut responsibilities, explicit rationing decisions are seldom taken and publicity about rationing and 'evidence based medicine' is hardly accessible to lay people. So, the conditions for publicity are not yet met.

In the case of public involvement, it is not clear who or what is 'the public'. If we mean citizens in the general sense, there is no evidence that they are eager to become involved in these types of decision making. At the same time, citizens seem to be quite aware of the existence of problems of choice in health care. As a result of the public campaigns and debates after the launch of the report of the Dunning Committee, a striking exception in the prevailing context of implicit decision making, public awareness has grown. Yet the Dutch government completely disregarded the results of these consultations (Tymstra and Andela 1993; Committee on Public Campaign Choices in Health Care 1995). In the paternalistic legacy of the former corporatist social relations of Dutch health care, there is apparently still no political danger in ignoring public consultations for priority setting (van der Grinten 2000).

Relevance

Since there is no real open debate and no properly organized exchange of arguments about the very issues of priority setting and rationing between all these stakeholders, it is hard to say if they can agree – we simply do not know. Yet we do have the strong tradition in Dutch health care of stakeholders inside and outside the government deliberating, negotiating and co-operating on a non-hierarchical basis, in order to end up with decisions that all fair-minded parties can agree. The future challenge is to explore sophisticated mechanisms of involvement and co-ordination, which encompass not only the 'rational' evidence and arguments but also the normative and value aspects of the very concrete questions of priority setting. A core problem, of course – and a core reason why the political process has such a poor track record in these matters – is the fact that it might be very hard to find solutions that 'all fair-minded parties' can agree to. In the end, we are dealing here with incomparable entities: weighing different types of suffering and potential remedies against each other; bridging the gap between individual stories of missed chances for a better life and tales of scarcity. In these conditions, it may be impossible to reach consensus – these are decisions that might remain essentially contestable.

Appeal

A distinction can be made between non-litigious and litigious appeals processes. There are no explicit appeal mechanisms in the Dutch health care system apart from the, mostly successful, political opposition in the parliament to the (proposed) removal of services from the insurance package (such as dental plates, the Pill, taxoids). There is no such thing as a national committee for priority setting. However, the general appeal mechanism (i.e. the law courts) is increasingly becoming the mechanism for challenging the (outcomes of) rationing policies. That makes sense in a system where citizens have rights by virtue of being insured for health care. They pay premiums for a defined package of care, either for compulsory or private insurance. Several people put on a waiting list for long-term care (nursing homes, home care) have recently successfully turned to the courts, which have declared the insurance organization (cure) and the government (care) as primarily responsible for delivering contracted services. It seems quite evident that these court judgments (and, in particular, the threat of future claims) will produce the climate for fundamental revisions of policies for priority setting and rationing.

Enforcement

As already explicated, enforcement mechanisms in Dutch health care are strongly influenced by the propensity to co-operate between the main stakeholders: government, providers of health care and insurers, especially at the meso and micro level of the system. There are some modest successes in involving professionals, service organizations and insurance companies in making choices in health care, but the public's voice is still not being properly heard.

THE FUTURE

With all this in mind, what of the different routes to health care technology decision making? How can we improve upon our current 'muddling through' while incorporating the well-founded critiques of overly rationalist approaches? One way of achieving cost reductions and quality control could be to pay much more attention to local efforts to streamline care, to create 'evidence based' care based not on 'universal' figures but on figures locally translated or collected (that are thus locally relevant and easier to gather). Based on local or regional information systems, indicators could be generated that are interpretable to local health care providers, and that can be fed back to them, thus stimulating them to constantly rethink their work and decision routines (Bates *et al.* 1999; Klazinga 2000).

   This, of course, is no grand solution to scarcity issues – but that is exactly the point. It is a means to attempt to reduce costs through local care innovations and arrangements in which insurers and patients may participate much more effectively than in large-scale, (inter)nationally driven attempts. Discussions about goals, values, and interpretations of data are also much more feasibly settled at the local level – if not through explicit discussion, then through an implicit understanding of the existing local needs and priorities. It is a means of putting professionals, with payers, in the lead in a more fruitful and creative way rather than as executors of some universal wisdom whose local validity is always contestable.

   Importantly, the word 'local' need not be taken merely to mean local geographically. As several authors have noted, working 'bottom up' from specialty-specific working groups, or co-ordinating efforts between MTA funders and professional guideline makers around specific topics (such as cholesterol medication) is much more feasible (Holm 1998). In this sense, we are not opting *against* the call for more information – but *for* more *relevant* information, more suitably circumscribed, to be used in the same contexts in which it was generated. This could consist of a carefully and modestly selected set of indicators (and not yet another 'comprehensive' but unfeasible wish list) used primarily by local health care professionals and managers – first and foremost for feedback, not control purposes. Such an approach would be in line with our insights elaborated above because there would be no attempt to transcend the diverse local projects with one common measure or criterion. QALYs, CEAs and guidelines would not lose their relevance – but their validity would not be stretched to breaking point by attempting to generalize between all too diverse contexts.

Yet strengthening such local efforts is not enough, in and by itself. We have argued that government cannot shy away from the responsibility to prioritize, and certainly not in the name of some 'technical' solution that would take away the need for difficult decisions. As Klein (1998: 960) has argued, 'in the absence of national decisions, equity is in danger' – and, we would add, professionals are put in an impossible bind. This, very sketchily, could lead us towards more 'polder model' bodies (involving patients, professionals, organizations, etc.) that are active in making such allocative (scarcity) decisions, at both the macro and meso level. We need such bodies to make decisions that have to be made but that cannot be resolved in a formal, rational, 'technical' way.

As Latour (1997) has argued, it is part and parcel of the nature of such political decisions that they are more about persuasion and conviction than about reason; that they are made under conditions of uncertainty and urgency that thwart any attempts to make them in a formally rational way; and that they are about relative distinctions between 'good' and 'bad' rather than searches for absolute grounds for such choices. In these decisions, the many layered 'costs' and 'effects' of new health care technologies should play a core role – and CEAs can be of help here in explicating at least some of these, and the normative considerations that abound here. Here again, then, the choice is not 'against' more information and 'for' new institutions: it is about making such information part and parcel of the political process rather than having it stand outside it, as an impersonal arbiter.[8]

We are not saying that these are easy solutions – at the very least, the past record of public decision making on these issues could make one rather pessimistic. Yet we argue that the currently prevalent alternatives – of delegating the hard choices to individual professionals or of pretending that we can solve these issues through technical means – are worse than the problem they are trying to solve. It is time to take up the challenge.

NOTES

1   The authors wish to thank Jannes Mulder, Els Grijseels, Niek Klazinga, Ashley Bloomfield, Norman Daniels, Chris Ham and Glenn Robert for their helpful comments.

2   Recently reframed to the independent Commission for Health Insurance (College voor Zorgverzekeringen).
3   For detailed discussions of the role of economic evaluations in Dutch health policy, see Elsinga and Rutten (1997) and Niessen *et al.* (2000).
4   This subsection is based on van der Grinten and Kasdorp (1999).
5   Most GP standards start with patients' symptoms, which makes the application of MTA very difficult. There are hardly any data available for such MTA analyses: studies rarely take a collection of symptoms as a starting point. This mismatch between the requirements of clinical practice and the clinical research set-up is an important problem for the utilization of MTA in clinical guidelines (cf. Berg *et al.* 2001).
6   Dutch CEA researchers argue that the change of emphasis in the evaluation of 'effectiveness' towards a longer-term perspective (life years gained, quality of life) is an important (and succesful) aim of their efforts (Grijseels, personal communication).
7   This section is based on van der Grinten and Kasdorp (1999).
8   More theoretically, this is not a choice between a 'scientific' and a 'political' way of solving these issues, but a fundamental search to *redefine* both categories so that they are no longer mutually exclusive (Latour 1997).

8

CONCLUSIONS
Chris Ham and Glenn Robert

In Chapter 2, we noted that from the late 1980s policy makers in a number of countries sought to set priorities for health care on a more explicit basis. The state of Oregon attracted most interest from policy analysts, but experience in the Netherlands, New Zealand, Norway and other systems was also widely reported and discussed. Research into comparative approaches to priority setting has identified three phases of development (Ham and Coulter 2001).

In the first phase, attention focused on the use of technical approaches to set priorities. These approaches included health technology assessment, cost–utility analysis, and epidemiological methods of health needs assessment. As Holm (1998) has noted, the emphasis placed on techniques reflected a belief that there was a right way to set priorities, drawing on the literature and research of a variety of disciplines, and harnessing the contribution of science and knowledge.

The second phase focused less on techniques than on decision making processes. This resulted from acknowledgement of the limits to science and also the role of values as well as evidence in decision making. Accordingly, policy makers sought to refine the methods used for determining health care priorities, both by involving experts and professionals in decision making, and by consulting organizations representing patients and the public.

The third phase of priority setting attempted to combine elements of the first two phases, recognizing that decisions needed to be based on sound techniques and on rigorous processes. As such, it rejected simple dichotomies, such as the debate between those who argued for more information to support decision making and those who contended that what were needed were stronger institutions to debate priorities (Klein and Williams 2000). Advocates of a synthesis of different approaches (Ham and Coulter 2001) started from the view that priority setting is an inherently messy and often political exercise and sought to strengthen both the evidence base of decisions and the processes through which these decisions are reached.

Underpinning many of the contributions to the literature in this field is recognition of the need for decision makers to be held to account for their decisions. The writings of Daniels and Sabin have been particularly important in this context in setting out the criteria that must be met to demonstrate accountability for reasonableness (Daniels and Sabin 1998). These criteria serve as a standard against which actual decisions may be assessed, as demonstrated by the contributors to this book.

In this final chapter, we bring together the findings from the country case studies to identify the emerging results. In so doing, the aim is to describe similarities and differences between countries and to summarize the state of the art of priority setting for health technologies. A further purpose is to take forward the debate about priority setting in the literature by assessing the lessons that can be drawn from practical experience. To what extent does priority setting in practice fulfil the criteria of accountability for reasonableness, and what does the experience of the countries studied here have to contribute to discussion of future directions in this field?

For ease of presentation, the chapter is organized around the seven questions that provided the framework for the authors in preparing their case studies.

1. WHAT PROCEDURES ARE USED TO DETERMINE WHETHER HEALTH TECHNOLOGIES SHOULD BE FUNDED?

In all countries, health technology assessment plays a part in determining whether technologies should be funded. This may involve the establishment of agencies charged with responsibility for undertaking assessments at a national or regional level; and these agencies may be constituted as institutions of government (as in Canada) or as non-governmental organizations (as in the Netherlands). The experience of New Zealand illustrates how policy makers have drawn on the results of health technology assessments in the case of a number of funding decisions (e.g. in relation to screening programmes).

Yet while all the authors highlight the role that health technology assessment plays in decision making, they also draw attention to its variable impact in practice. Obstacles to the use of health technology assessment include the limited understanding of its contribution among policy makers, the gap between the demand for evidence based assessments and the ability of researchers to meet that demand, and the many other influences on decision making. As a consequence, health technology assessment is rarely the only or the main factor taken into account by decision makers.

One of the reasons for this is that the agencies that undertake health technology assessments are usually advisory in nature. This means that even when assessments are undertaken, policy makers in health ministries retain discretion over whether to accept the results and the advice offered. Also, only a small proportion of health technologies are subject to assessment before their introduction into practice.

For the majority of technologies that do not go through an assessment process, pressure from interested organizations, the advice of experts and the judgement of decision makers hold the key to determining whether technologies should be funded. As the Canadian case illustrates, this often means committees of professional and lay members having to weigh whatever evidence is available, and to factor in the values they consider relevant. And as the Norwegian case shows, it may be difficult to understand the basis of decision making in such committees, given that priority setting at the meso and micro levels is often less visible to researchers (a conclusion reinforced by the Dutch and UK cases).

2. WHAT IS THE ROLE OF DIFFERENT INSTITUTIONS IN THESE PROCEDURES?

In all countries, priority setting occurs at different levels. At the macro level, the evidence reported here indicates that it is uncommon for a single agency to have sole responsibility for priority setting. In this respect, the UK is unusual in having created a new institution, the National Institute for Clinical Excellence (NICE), with an explicit remit to advise on the funding of health technologies. To be sure, other agencies are also involved in work on setting priorities in the UK, but since 1999 NICE has been the focus for much of the work in this area.

The other countries studied have a greater degree of institutional pluralism. This is illustrated by New Zealand, which, despite its small size, relies on the work of the National Health Committee, the Health Funding Authority (until recently) and PHARMAC, as well as New Zealand Health Technology Assessment and *ad hoc* expert groups. Similarly, in the Netherlands there exists what Berg and van der Grinten describe as 'a patchy assembly of rather different approaches . . . and institutions' charged with responsibility for priority setting. Lack of co-ordination between these institutions is emphasized by Berg and van der Grinten in their analysis.

Another point to emerge from the Dutch case is the shift of focus after the Dunning Report from the macro level to the meso and micro levels. A similar observation is made by Norheim about Norway, where the two reports from the Lønning Commission at a national level have attracted international interest but where decision making on priorities continues to be focused on the county councils. In this context, the Canadian case is of particular interest because of its analysis of the meso level in relation to cancer and cardiac services. The authors show how the committees responsible for priority setting went about this task, drawing on a combination of evidence and values in the process.

Institutional pluralism, combined with a blurring of roles between different levels, enables decision makers to shift responsibility and blame for difficult and unpopular choices. In this sense, lack of clarity serves an important political function in making accountability for decisions difficult to pin down. This helps to explain why some systems have avoided clarifying the roles of different actors and institutions in relation to priority setting. The ability to shift blame and fudge accountability also accounts for the retreat from explicit approaches to priority setting at a macro level in those systems (like New Zealand and the Netherlands) that flirted with such approaches in the early 1990s. Similarly, Norway has avoided focusing responsibility on a single agency, and Norheim notes that as a consequence it is 'difficult to identify institutions where such [priority setting] decisions take place'.

It remains to be seen what will happen in the UK, which came to explicitness relatively late in the day and which is in the early stages of testing the contribution of NICE and its implications for accountability. The establishment of an institution operating at arm's length from government may insulate policy makers from the effects of priority setting decisions, although this depends on the willingness of politicians to allow NICE sufficient freedom of action to preserve its independence. It should also be noted that health authorities are not required to follow NICE guidance (Newdick 2001), creating the possibility that the postcode lottery that NICE was intended to eliminate will continue.

3. WHAT KIND OF EVIDENCE DO THESE INSTITUTIONS EXPECT/REQUIRE/CONSIDER IN MAKING FUNDING DECISIONS?

The cases reported here indicate that evidence from clinical trials and research studies provides the main basis for priority setting decisions. Such evidence may be drawn from randomized controlled trials where available, and other sources where evidence of this standard is lacking. Systematic reviews and meta-analyses of separate studies are reported to be used in a number of countries. Evidence on the costs of technologies and cost-effectiveness are also seen as relevant, although usually as a supplement to information from clinical sources rather than as a determining factor in itself.

Alongside scientific evidence, a range of other information may be accessed by decision makers. In New Zealand, for example, the impact of decisions on Maori health is an essential component of decision making, and input from Maori as well as Pacific Island and consumer representatives is routinely sought. More generally, the case studies show that decision makers have acknowledged the need to take account of a variety of values in their work. These values include not only health benefit for patients (as demonstrated by studies of clinical and cost effectiveness) but also equity and social acceptability. Having made this point, the methods for assessing clinical and cost effectiveness are more advanced (though still incomplete) in their development than the methods for analysing the impact on equity and social acceptability.

This is where institutional innovations like the NICE Citizens Council in the UK may contain clues as to the means by which decision making procedures can be strengthened to incorporate a range of values. The role of the Council, established in 2002, is to bring lay perspectives to bear on priority setting decisions. Other countries such as New Zealand and the Netherlands have also experimented with various forms of public involvement in priority setting, while the Canadian case, reported here and elsewhere (Singer *et al.* 2000), illustrates the role that lay members of priority setting committees can play. What is now needed is to assess the contribution of these different mechanisms in enabling decision makers to arrive at judgements on the use of resources. As this happens, there is a cautionary tale from the Netherlands where the results of public consultation were ignored by decision makers (Berg and van der Grinten, this book).

4. WHAT STANDARD OF PROOF DO INSTITUTIONS EXPECT TO BE DEMONSTRATED IN AGREEING FUNDING?

The idea that decisions on priorities should be subject to a standard of proof was first proposed by Hadhorn in his analysis of the parallels between medical and legal decision making (Hadhorn 1992). He argued that just as legal decisions depended on the available evidence, so too medical decisions might be expected to meet a standard of proof before agreement was given that treatment should proceed. The stringency of the standard could, in Hadhorn's view, be higher or lower, depending on the seriousness of the medical condition in question and the consequence of not intervening, and might require that significant net health benefit is established before funding is agreed. As he notes,

> the choice of a standard for defining health care needs to reflect society's values. Indeed, it is here, in the selection of the standard of proof, that the fundamental balance between individual claims of need (that is, pursuit of individual good) and the greater public good is achieved.
>
> (Hadhorn 1992: 93)

Although not using this phraseology, the Dunning Report in the Netherlands was arguably an attempt to apply a standard of proof to decisions on what should be included in the health insurance basket. The report proposed that four tests should be applied in arriving at coverage decisions: whether the care was necessary from the community's point of view; effective; efficient; and could be left to individuals to fund directly. A similar approach was adopted by the National Health Committee in New Zealand. In its work, the Committee made use of four principles in deciding whether services should be funded: the treatment or service should provide benefit (effectiveness); value for money (efficiency); be a fair use of public money (equity); and be consistent with communities' values (acceptability). Also in New Zealand, PHARMAC requires that the evidence demonstrates 'significant and cost-effective health gain' before agreeing to funding of new drugs.

In practice, neither the Netherlands nor New Zealand developed these broad templates in a way that could easily be applied in decision making. They also decided not to set priorities mainly by excluding technologies from coverage. Rather, they used evidence from clinical trials and other studies to draw up guidelines on priorities. As Bloomfield notes, the standard of proof required in New Zealand in arriving at these decisions is generally high, drawing on randomized controlled trials and other rigorous evidence where possible. Not only this, but also decisions on pharmaceutical coverage have drawn on cost–utility analysis.

There are parallels here with UK experience. The attention given to NICE and its public method of operation creates a strong incentive to demonstrate that decisions are based on evidence and that the reasons for these decisions are explained. In its early work, NICE has relied extensively on evidence on clinical effectiveness and has in a small number of cases advised against the funding of new technologies where the evidence is weak. It has also made some use of cost–utility analysis, although at this stage only in relation to individual technologies rather than in making comparative judgements. In so doing, NICE has seemingly adopted an implicit standard that a technology should not be recommended for funding if the cost per quality-adjusted life year exceeds £30,000 (McDonald 2001). The general absence of comparative information has left local commissioners of health care with the difficult task of implementing NICE guidance without any overall framework for determining which of these new technologies are the 'best buy' for their population.

In Norway, the standard of proof required is implicit except in the case of cancer services. As Norheim shows, new technologies are compared with standard treatment for cancer using the following criteria:

1. Treatment aiming for cure: 5–10 per cent absolute improvement in long-term survival (usually measured as five-year survival).
2. Treatment aiming for extended time to live: median survival improved by at least 20 per cent or minimum three months.
3. Treatment aiming for prevention of symptoms related to cancer: no minimum standard is defined, because there is no consensus on the relevant clinical endpoints.
4. Treatment intended for relief of symptoms: more than 20 per cent of the patients must have improvement of subjective symptoms such as pain, nausea, heavy breathing or other complaints.

In emphasizing the use of evidence and standards of proof, it would be wrong to give the impression that decision making is invariably driven by rational methods. As we have already noted, in all countries reviewed there are examples of policy makers responding to political pressure rather than the claims of evidence and agreeing to fund health technologies even when the scientific basis is weak. This was illustrated in New Zealand in relation to the funding of hepatitis B screening. The funding of this screening programme was agreed even though planning was well advanced for a pilot programme and the Ministry of Health and other funders were opposed to national implementation (Bloomfield, this book). A different example comes from the Netherlands, where the evidence on the effectiveness of Viagra was ignored by policy makers who decided not to fund this drug even though a technology assessment had demonstrated its cost-effectiveness (Berg and van der Grinten, this book).

5. WHAT APPEAL MECHANISMS ARE AVAILABLE FOR REVIEWING DECISIONS?

The evidence reported in this book indicates that there are three main types of appeal mechanism in place. First, there are formal mechanisms related to specific types of decision. This is exemplified in Norway in the existence of an independent appeal board dealing with treatment abroad. As Norheim notes, the board is a kind of administrative 'court' chaired by a judge and with four members including doctors, representatives from health service administration and patient organizations, and a medical ethicist. During its first three years, the appeal board considered 184 decisions, and 21 of these were reversed.

Another example of a formal mechanism is the appeal panel used by NICE in the UK. Manufacturers or sponsors of technologies who object to a NICE decision, as well as others with a genuine interest in the subject matter, have ten days to make an appeal which is heard by a panel made up of three non-executive members of NICE and two independent members. As Robert shows, the main basis for an appeal is on the grounds of procedural fairness, although decisions that appear perverse in the light of evidence may also be contested. An example was the appeal against the decision on the use of paclitaxel in the second-line treatment of breast cancer that was upheld in 2000. On the other hand, appeals against the determinations on zanamivir and hip prostheses were rejected.

The second type of appeal mechanism is the courts. Legal challenges are a feature of priority setting in all countries, as illustrated in New Zealand in the case of patients denied treatment and decisions on the funding of pharmaceuticals. As Bloomfield shows, pharmaceutical companies have resorted to litigation on a number of occasions, in one instance taking a case as far as the Privy Council. Almost all cases have been defended successfully. Action by pharmaceutical companies in the courts has also occurred in Canada.

The courts have also been invoked in the Netherlands, the only system in our study where insurance is the main form of funding. Berg and van der Grinten note the absence in the Netherlands of formal appeal mechanisms as in Norway and the UK. As they comment, 'the general appeal mechanism (i.e. the law courts) is increasingly becoming the mechanism for challenging the (outcomes of) rationing policies'. Patients have used the courts to secure access to treatment and care, and this in turn has influenced the climate in which priority setting decisions are taken.

The third type of appeal mechanism is lobbying and the use of the media and other sources to highlight grievances and to seek to reverse decisions. There is evidence of this from all countries. For example, in the Netherlands a proposal to exclude contraceptives from funding in the health insurance package was withdrawn following protests by women's organizations and family planning groups. In New Zealand, the media has been used by the families of two patients denied access to dialysis treatment, and in one of these cases the decision was changed on review. The same applied in Norway in the Sandberg and Matheson cases and in the UK in the Child B case. And in Canada the government committed more funds to radiation therapy after media pressure highlighted the difficulties faced by Ontario patients who were sent to the United States to receive treatment when waiting lists became unacceptably long.

6. WHAT DOES EXPERIENCE SAY ABOUT THE DEBATE BETWEEN THOSE WHO ARGUE FOR STRONGER INSTITUTIONS AND THOSE WHO ARGUE FOR BETTER INFORMATION TO SUPPORT PRIORITY SETTING?

The evidence we have reviewed demonstrates a continuing process of institutional innovation in priority setting alongside an investment in information to support decision making. Taking information first, the interest shown in health technology assessment and evidence based medicine has spawned both national and international efforts to strengthen the information base available to decision makers. In Canada, this is exemplified by the setting up of the Canadian Institute for Health Information charged with identifying health information needs, collecting, processing and maintaining data, and related functions.

In the UK there has been a sizeable investment in information through government support for research into the clinical and cost effectiveness of health technologies. This includes funding of the Cochrane Centre at Oxford and the Centre for Reviews and Dissemination at York, alongside a research and development programme on health technology assessment. There are parallels here with the Netherlands, with a mixture of government and private funding supporting efforts to evaluate health technologies. These national efforts are increasingly linked through international networks such as the Cochrane Collaboration.

Turning to institutions, there are examples of innovation in all countries and at different levels. At the macro level, the responsibility given to organizations such as the National Health Committee and the Health Funding Authority in New Zealand and NICE in the UK is symptomatic of the attempt by policy makers to find better ways of using information and evidence in decision making. Much the same applies in Norway with the recent establishment of a Centre for Health Technology Assessment.

At the meso level, the use in Canada of committees to set priorities for cancer care and cardiac services in Ontario illustrates the interest shown in that country in new institutional forms. There are parallels here with both New Zealand, where the newly created district health boards will be involved in priority setting at the meso level, and the UK, where health authorities have set up priorities forums and similar mechanisms to assist in decision making.

The case of the Netherlands highlights a further point, namely the part played by medical bodies in priority setting. As Berg and van der Grinten demonstrate, the focus of priority setting in the Netherlands has shifted back from the macro to the meso and micro levels. In the process, greater emphasis has been placed on the use of guidelines as a priority setting tool. Medical organizations have been closely involved in the work done on guidelines. The same applies in New Zealand, where guidelines have also been given prominence and where clinicians have been extensively involved in the development of priority access criteria in relation to waiting lists. The UK has also invested in the development of guidelines through NICE and other mechanisms.

Partly as a consequence, there is a large and growing literature on the role of guidelines in clinical decision making (Grol 1997; Haycox *et al.* 1999; Woolf *et al.* 1999). This literature has highlighted not only the benefits of guidelines but also the potential harms, the latter including their inflexibility and inability to offer individualized care for patients with special needs. Guidelines may curtail the discretion of clinicians and they may also pre-empt resources by advocating the uptake of expensive new technologies. This has led some authors to argue that less emphasis should be placed on guidelines and more on other means of improving the utilization of resources and outcomes, such as audit and continuing professional education. It should also be noted that doctors may not follow clinical guidelines, and a review of the literature has identified the reasons for this (Cabana *et al.* 1999).

The institutional innovations in the field of rationing have advanced the use of techniques and scientific evidence in decision making. There has been less progress to date in finding effective ways of involving patients' organizations and the public. In Canada, lay input is channelled mainly through membership of priority setting committees, and in New Zealand there have been various efforts to involve consumers and consumer organizations in work on guidelines and priority setting as a whole. Only in the UK, with the Citizens Council set up to advise NICE on priority setting, has a specific institutional initiative designed to facilitate public involvement been taken. While it is too early to comment on the work of the Council, the decision to establish such a body to advise NICE is in itself an indication of the importance policy makers are attaching to widening the basis of participation in decision making.

7. TO WHAT EXTENT DOES EXPERIENCE MEET THE TESTS OF ACCOUNTABILITY FOR REASONABLENESS?

We will discuss in turn each of Daniels and Sabin's tests of accountability for reasonableness in relation to priority setting decisions.

Publicity

The evidence on this point indicates wide variation in practice. At one extreme are countries like Canada, the Netherlands and

Norway, where the publicity condition is usually not met. At the other are New Zealand and the UK, where decisions are increasingly accessible to the public. Yet even in these more open systems there are restrictions on the availability of information, as illustrated by lack of transparency in the private sector in New Zealand, and the constraints of a 'commercial in confidence' culture in the case of some of NICE's decisions. Not only this, but also priority setting decisions that fall outside the ambit of institutions such as NICE in the UK may be just as opaque as those that are taken in other countries.

Relevance

Variations in publicity and transparency directly influence the extent to which the relevance condition is met. By definition, where there is no or limited publicity, it is difficult if not impossible to establish the relevance of the rationales used in decision making.

As an example, in the Netherlands, the current emphasis on decisions at the meso and micro levels means that priority setting is mainly implicit and the rationales are not available for public scrutiny. There is somewhat greater openness in Canada in areas like cancer and cardiac care, but with these exceptions there is no basis on which to assess compliance with the relevance condition. Much the same applies in Norway.

New Zealand and the UK again offer contrasting experience. Bloomfield argues on the basis of his review that the rationales used in New Zealand do generally rest on evidence that fair-minded parties can agree are relevant. Similarly, Robert shows that the use by NICE of criteria such as clinical effectiveness, cost-effectiveness, and the wider implications of decisions fulfils the conditions set out by Daniels and Sabin in this area. The decisions of NICE may still be contentious, but the application of these criteria is generally accepted as being appropriate by different stakeholders.

Appeals

As noted above, there are different types of appeal mechanism. In the context of Daniels and Sabin's framework, it is the formal appeals mechanisms, rather than the courts and political lobbying, that are relevant to this discussion.

Only Norway and the UK have established such mechanisms

to date. In Norway, they take two forms: the appeal board that considers cases for treatment abroad (discussed earlier) at the macro level; and the hearings used at the meso level to consider clinical guidelines. Although not strictly formal appeals, these hearings enable challenges to guidelines to be heard and offer the opportunity for revisions to be made.

In the UK, NICE has developed a formal appeal mechanism that has been used on a number of occasions. This has resulted in revisions to decisions in some cases and confirmation of decisions in others. NICE is also willing to review earlier decisions in the light of new evidence, as in the case of Relenza, where a decision to not recommend funding was changed following the presentation of fresh data.

Enforcement

The fourth and final condition on enforcement is not met anywhere. Given that the UK, through NICE, offers the closest approximation to the accountability for reasonableness tests, it is in that country that effective enforcement is most likely to be found. In practice, enforcement in the UK is informal and voluntary, relying first and foremost on the integrity of NICE itself and government oversight, with, in the background, the threat of legal action by aggrieved stakeholders should NICE fail to observe due process in decision making. In addition, Parliamentary scrutiny is provided through the Health Select Committee which includes members from across the various political parties. NICE has been a topic for inquiry by the Committee in February 1999 and again in February 2002. Select committees are appointed by Parliament to scrutinize the work of government departments, and their findings and recommendations are submitted to Parliament. Inquiries like those undertaken into the work of NICE represent a form of regulation and help to ensure that the methods used by NICE are rigorous and defensible.

In other countries, the threat of legal challenge and judicial review of decisions similarly acts as a spur to decision makers to adopt rigorous and fair procedures, given the prospect that they may be required to defend their decisions in the courts. This kind of legal regulation does, however, fall outside the categories of voluntary or public regulation envisaged by Daniels and Sabin in articulating the accountability for reasonableness criteria.

CONCLUSIONS

To return to the starting point of this chapter, the evidence we have summarized and analysed underlines arguments developed elsewhere on priority setting as both a political process and an exercise in policy learning (Chapter 2, this book). The politics of priority setting is demonstrated by the lobbying associated with decisions on the funding of technologies and the willingness of politicians to shift responsibility and blame to others for difficult and unpopular decisions (cf. the Netherlands case). It is also evident in the willingness of politicians to make or change decisions even when the scientific evidence points in the opposite direction (cf. New Zealand and Norway). To this extent, priority setting is no different from other areas of health policy, even though the rhetoric of evidence based medicine and the scientific basis of health care might suggest otherwise.

The policy learning associated with priority setting is demonstrated in a variety of ways. An example is the retreat from explicit approaches at the macro level in the Netherlands in the face of the political costs involved. A further example is the strengthening of the information base to support priority setting, for which there is evidence in all countries. Particularly striking is the learning that has arisen in relation to the institutional basis of decision making, with a wide variety of different committees and organizations being established at different levels to provide the focus for priority setting work.

The outstanding question is what the evidence reviewed here has to say about the state of the art of priority setting and the prospects for the third phase of work in this area, with its emphasis on techniques as well as processes. Our own assessment is that there remains considerable scope for strengthening both the information base to support decision making and the institutions charged with responsibility for setting priorities. While examples of innovation and emerging good practice can be found in all countries, overall there remains a distance to travel before the requirements of accountability for reasonableness are met.

To be more concrete, there is a need for greater openness in decision making, a stronger commitment to giving reasons for decisions, the development of formal appeal mechanisms, and regulation of the decision making process. In parallel, there is scope for involving patients' organizations and the public in priority setting in recognition of the role that values play in decision making and the need for decision makers to demonstrate legitimacy to different stakeholders. More broadly, by involving these organizations, there is an opportunity to enhance democratic deliberation in priority setting and in the process open up the ethical dilemmas that underpin choices in health care.

The gap between these aspirations and current reality raises the question why this should be so. One is that the rationalist assumptions underpinning accountability for reasonableness may conflict with the politics of priority setting. Publicity and giving reasons for decisions leave decision makers open to criticism and challenge in a way that being implicit and muddling through do not. It is partly for this reason that there has been no linear progression from implicit to explicit approaches. Indeed, it has been suggested that the interest in explicit priority setting at a macro level that began to emerge in the late 1980s may, with the benefit of hindsight, be seen as a temporary aberration in a much longer tradition of blame avoidance and incrementalism (Chapter 2, this book).

Partly because of this, long-established rationing tools such as waiting lists continue to play an important part in reconciling rising demands and constrained resources. In all of the countries whose experiences have been reviewed here, waiting lists for non-urgent treatment present a challenge to policy makers seeking to improve health system performance. New Zealand has focused particularly on the development of priority-scoring criteria in the management of waiting lists, and some of the experience gained in New Zealand has been adapted in Canada in the Western Canadian Waiting List project. By contrast, Norway and the UK have sought to set targets for the reduction of waiting lists and waiting times without using explicit criteria to determine who should receive priority in the queue. In the Netherlands, the attempt by companies to obtain quicker access to treatment for their employees by bypassing traditional waiting lists stimulated a debate about equity in that country and resulted in action to ban preferential treatment for employees.

Another reason for the gap between aspiration and reality is that the issues involved in priority setting are inherently difficult and contested. Achieving consensus on either outcomes or process has been a challenge in all systems, and the experience reviewed here testifies to the efforts made by policy makers to find a way forward in territory that remains controversial. In these circumstances, the requirements of accountability for reasonableness may be too demanding, and the claims of those who favour implicit priority setting may carry the day. In this context, the arguments of the implicit rationers, first articulated by Calabresi and Bobbit (1978), continue to be argued with force (Mechanic 1997).

Our own view is that while these arguments are important, they are less compelling than the case for being more explicit and consistent. The combined effects of a more informed and demanding public, a media that scrutinizes health services' decision making ever more intensely, and a legal profession willing to challenge medical judgements means that those who favour implicit approaches risk finding themselves on the wrong side of history. Not only this, but also opening up decision making offers an opportunity to engage in the process of social learning about the limits to medicine and the need to make choices in health care (Daniels and Sabin 2002), provided that appropriate mechanisms and institutions are in place. This process needs to take place at the macro level in relation to the responsibilities of government, at the meso level in relation to the choices made by health authorities and similar bodies, and at the micro level, as when doctors and patients engage in shared decision making.

Our final point returns to address the debate between the advocates of more information and stronger institutions to support priority setting. Based on the work reported here, it is evident that the establishment of new institutions creates an appetite for information to enable these institutions to carry out their remit. This has certainly been the case in the UK, where NICE has proved itself to be information-hungry and has created a demand for data on clinical and cost effectiveness that has been difficult to satisfy. In this sense, commentators such as Williams and Klein may yet be able to find common cause in that institutions require information, while information needs an institutional context in which to be debated and applied. What this suggests is that strengthening the institutional framework for priority setting is likely to increase the demand for and use of information, whether or not this is planned. And as effort is put into increasing the role of the public in priority setting, this information will increasingly encompass data about social preferences as well as evidence of clinical and cost effectiveness.

REFERENCES

Åbyholm, G., Riise, G., Melsom, M.N., Piene, H. and Gulbrandsen, I. (1997) Ventetidsgarantien og garantibrudd, *Tidsskrift for den Norske Lægeforening*, 117(3): 366–8.

Association of the British Pharmaceutical Industry (1999) *NICE and Medicines*, BSC/6/99/4K. London: ABPI.

Baron, J. (1995) Blind justice: Fairness in groups and the do-no-harm principle, *Journal of Behavior and Decision Making*, 8: 71–83.

Barrett, B.J., Parfrey, P.S., Foley, R.N. and Detsky, A.S. (1994) An economic analysis of strategies for the use of contrast media for diagnostic cardiac catheterization, *Medical Decision Making*, 14(4): 325–35.

Barrett, B.J., Parfrey, P.S. and Morton, B.C. (1998) Safety and criteria for selective use of low-osmolarity contrast for cardiac angiography, *Medical Care*, 36(8): 1189–97.

Bates, D.W., Pappius, E., Kuperman, G.J. *et al.* (1999) Using information systems to measure and improve quality, *International Journal of Medical Informatics*, 53: 115–24.

Battista, R.N. (1996) Towards a paradigm for technology assessment, in M. Peckam and R. Smith (eds) *Scientific Basis of Health Services*. London: BMJ Publishing Group.

Battista, R.N. and Hodge, M.J. (1999) The evolving paradigm of health technology assessment: reflections for the millennium, *Canadian Medical Association Journal*, 160: 1464–7.

Battista, R.N., Hodge, M.J. and Vineis, P. (1995) Medicine, practice and guidelines: the uneasy juncture of science and art, *Journal of Clinical Epidemiology*, 48: 875–80.

Beecham, L. (2000) Health Secretary sets out NICE's programme, *British Medical Journal*, 320: 63.

Berg, M., ter Meulen, R.H.J. and van der Burg, M. (2001) Guidelines for appropriate care: the importance of empirical normative analysis, *Health Care Analysis*, 9: 77–99.

Bezwoda, W.R., Seymour, L. and Dansey, R.D. (1995) High-dose chemotherapy with hematopoietic rescue as primary treatment for metastatic breast cancer: a randomized trial, *Journal of Clinical Oncology*, 13(10): 2483–9.

Bjørndal, A. and Guldvog, B. (1996) Venteliste til besvær, *Tidsskrift for den Norske Lægeforening*, 116(8): 943–4.

Blakely, T. and Thornley, C. (1999) Screening for hepatitis B carriers: evidence and policy development in New Zealand, *New Zealand Medical Journal*, 112: 431–3.

Bloor, K., Freemantle, N., Khadjesari, Z. and Maynard, A. (2003) Impact of NICE guidance on laparoscopic surgery for inguinal hernias: analysis of interrupted time series, *British Medical Journal*, 326: 578.

Bodenheimer, T. (1997) The Oregon Health Plan: lessons for the nation, *New England Journal of Medicine*, 337: 651–6, 720–3.

Boer, A. (1999) Assessment and regulation of health care technology. The Dutch experience, *International Journal of Technology Assessment in Health Care*, 15: 638–48.

Borst-Eilers, E. (1998). Keynote address. Paper presented to the Second International Conference on Priorities in Health Care, London.

Borud, H. (1996a) Hernes overprøver ekspertene, *Aftenposten*, 13 July.

Borud, H. (1996b) Kreftleger raser mot Hernes, *Aftenposten*, 14 July.

Borud, H. (1996c) Krefteksperter går i protest, *Aftenposten*, 14 July.

Boseley, S. (2000) GPs rebel against flu drug advice, *The Guardian*, 11 December.

Bowling, A., Jacobson, B. and Southgate, L. (1993) Explorations in consultation of the public and health professionals on priority setting in an inner London health district, *Social Science and Medicine*, 37: 851–7.

Brinch, L., Evensen, S.A., Blomhoff, J.P. and Albrechtsen, D. (1993) Tenke det, ville det, og så gjøre det, *Tidsskrift for den Norske Lægeforening*, 113(27): 3392–4.

Browne, A. (2000) GPs warned as they snub advice on anti-flu drug, *The Observer*, 10 December.

Burke, K. (2002a) NICE accuses drug companies of withholding data, *British Medical Journal*, 324: 320.

Burke, K. (2002b) No cash to implement NICE, health authorities tell MPs, *British Medical Journal*, 324: 258.

Burke, K. (2002c) NICE may fail to stop 'postcode prescribing', MPs told, *British Medical Journal*, 324: 191.

Buxton, M. (1999) How will NICE impact on the use of new and existing technologies in the NHS. Paper presented to the 'priority setting in the NHS' conference, London, 21 September.

Cabana, M., Rand, C., Powe, N. *et al.* (1999) Why don't physicians follow clinical practice guidelines? *Journal of the American Medical Association*, 282(15): 1458–65.

Calabresi, G. and Bobbit, P. (1978) *Tragic Choices*. New York: Norton.

Canadian Coordinating Office for Health Technology Assessment (1995) (brochure). Ottawa: CCOHTA.

Canadian Institute for Health Information (2000) *Health Care in Canada 2000: A First Annual Report* (website: httpl//secure.cihi.ca/cihiweb/products/Healthreport 2000.pdf)

Chinitz, D., Shalev, C., Galai, N. and Israeli, A. (1998) Israel's basic basket of health services: the importance of being explicitly implicit, *British Medical Journal*, 317: 1005–7.

Collier, J. (1998) Drug and Therapeutics Bulletin defends its stance over donepezil, *British Medical Journal*, 316(7137): 1092.

Committee on Choices in Health Care (1992) *Choices in Health Care.* Rijswijk: Ministry of Welfare, Health and Cultural Affairs.

Committee on Public Campaign Choices in Health Care (1995) Keuzen in de Gezondheidszorg. Verslag van de vierjatige Publiekscampagne Keuzen in de Zorg. The Hague: Ministry of Health, Welfare and Sports.

Conseil d'Évaluation des Technologies de la Santé (CETS) (1990) *Evaluation of Low versus High Osmolar Contrast Media.* Montreal: CETS.

Cookson, R. and Dolan, P. (1999) Public views on health care rationing: a group discussion study, *Health Policy*, 49: 63–74.

Cookson, R., McDaid, D. and Maynard, A. (2001) Wrong SIGN, NICE mess: is national guidance distorting allocation of resources? *British Medical Journal*, 323: 743–5.

Coulter, A. (1999) NICE and CHI: reducing variations and raising standards, in J. Appleby and A. Harrison (eds) *Health Care UK 1999/ 2000. The King's Fund Review of Health Policy*. London: King's Fund.

Coulter, A. and Ham, C. (eds) (2000) *The Global Challenge of Health Care Rationing*. Buckingham: Open University Press.

Cowper, A. (2002) NICE: still advancing the excellence curve, *British Journal of Healthcare Management*, 8(3): 92–5.

Daniels, N. (1994) Four unsolved rationing problems. A challenge, *Hastings Center Report*, 24(4): 27–9.

Daniels, N. (2000) Accountability for reasonableness, *British Medical Journal*, 321: 1300–1.

Daniels, N. and Sabin, J. (1997) Limits to health care: Fair procedures, democratic deliberation, and the legitimacy problem for insurers, *Philosophy and Public Affairs*, 4: 303–50.

Daniels, N. and Sabin, J. (1998a) The ethics of accountability in managed care reform, *Health Affairs*, 17: 50–63.

Daniels, N. and Sabin, J. (2002) *Setting Limits Fairly: Can We Learn to Share Medical Resources?* Oxford: Oxford University Press.

Day, P. and Klein, R. (1998). The dilemmas of choice, *Odyssey*, 4: 8–13.

Deber, R.B. and Goel, V. (1990) Using explicit decision rules to manage issues of justice, risk, and ethics in decision analysis: when is it not rational to maximize expected utility? *Medical Decision Making*, 10: 181–94.

Deber, R., Wiktorowicz, M., Leatt, P. and Champagne, F. (1994) Technology acquisition in Canadian hospitals: How is it done, and where is the information coming from? *Healthcare Management Forum*, 7(4): 18–27.

Dent, T. and Sadler, M. (2002) From guidance to practice: why NICE is not enough, *British Medical Journal*, 324: 842–5.

Department of Health (1997) *The New NHS: Modern, Dependable*, Cm. 3807. London: The Stationery Office.

Department of Health (1998) *A First Class Service: Quality in the New NHS*. London: Department of Health.

Detsky, A. (1993) Guidelines for economic analysis of pharmaceutical products: a draft document for Ontario and Canada, *Pharmacoeconomics*, 3(5): 354–61.

Dewar, S. (1999) Viagra: the political management of rationing, in J. Appleby and A. Harrison (eds) *Health Care UK. The King's Fund Review of Health Policy*. London: King's Fund.

Dillon, A. (2002) Opening the doors on NICE: the next steps, *British Journal of Healthcare Management*, 8(3): 96–7.

Dodds-Smith, I. (2000) NICE and the ultimate decision makers: the legal framework for prescription and reimbursement of medicines, in A. Miles, J.R. Hampton and B. Hurwitz (eds) *NICE, CHI and the NHS Reforms. Enabling Excellence or Imposing Control?* London: Aesculapius Medical Press.

D'Souza, D., Martin, D.K., Purdy, L., Bezjak, A. and Singer, P.A. (2001) The waiting list for radiation therapy: A case study, *BMC Health Services Research*, 1: 3.

Eaton, L. (2000) A dose of scepticism, *Health Services Journal*, 20 July.

Eddy, D.M. (1991) Oregon's methods: did cost-effectiveness analysis fail? *Journal of the American Medical Association*, 266: 2135–41.

Eddy, D.M. (1994) Principles for making difficult decisions in difficult times, *Journal of the American Medical Association*, 271: 792–8.

Eddy, D.M. (1996) Benefit language: criteria that will improve quality while reducing costs, *Journal of the American Medical Association*, 275: 650–7.

Edgar, W. (2000) Rationing health care in New Zealand – how the public has a say, in A. Coulter and C. Ham (eds) *The Global Challenge of Health Care Rationing*. Buckingham: Open University Press.

Ellis, S.J. (1999) Fidelity and stewardship are incompatible when attempted by same individual, *British Medical Journal*, 318: 940.

Elsinga, E. and Rutten, F.F.H. (1997) Economic evaluation in support of national health policy: the case of the Netherlands, *Social Science and Medicine*, 45: 605–20.

European Observatory on Health Care Systems (2000) *Health Care Systems in Transition: Norway*, Report No. AMS 5012667 (NOR). Copenhagen: EOHCS.

Executive Committee of the World Marrow Donor Association (1992) Bone marrow transplants using volunteer donors – recommendations and requirements for a standardized practice throughout the world, *Bone Marrow Transplantation*, 10: 287–91.

Feek, C.M., McKean, W., Henneveld, L. *et al.* (1999) Experience with rationing health care in New Zealand, *British Medical Journal*, 318: 1346–8.

Ferriman, A. (2000) Milburn to monitor implementation of NICE guidance, *British Medical Journal*, 321: 1431.

Fleck, L.M. (1992) Just healthcare rationing: a democratic decision making approach, *University of Pennsylvania Law Review*, 140(5): 1597–636.

Freemantle, N. (2000) Valuing the effects of sildenafil in erectile dysfunction. Strong assumptions are required to generate a QALY value, *British Medical Journal*, 320: 1156–7.

Giacomini, M.K. (1999) The which-hunt: assembling health technologies for assessment and rationing, *Journal of Health Politics, Policy and Law*, 24(4): 715–58.

Goel, V., Deber, R.B. and Detsky, A.S. (1989) Nonionic contrast media: economic analysis and health policy development, *Canadian Medical Association Journal*, 140(4): 389–95.

Greenhalgh, T. (1997) Advertisements for donepezil. More convincing evidence of efficacy needs to be cited, *British Medical Journal*, 315: 1623.

Grimshaw, J., Freemantle, N., Wallace, S. *et al.* (1995) Developing and implementing clinical practice guidelines, *Quality in Health Care*, 4: 55–64.

Grol, R. (1997) Beliefs and evidence in changing clinical practice, *British Medical Journal*, 315: 418–21.

Hadhorn, D. (1991) Setting health care priorities in Oregon. Cost effectiveness meets the rule of rescue, *Journal of the American Medical Association*, 265: 2218–25.

Hadhorn, D. (1992) Emerging parallels in the American health care and legal-judicial systems, *American Journal of Law and Medicine*, XVIII: 73–96.

Hadhorn, D. and Holmes, A.C. (1997a) The New Zealand priority criteria project. Part 1: Overview, *British Medical Journal*, 314: 131–4.

Hadhorn, D. and Holmes, A.C. (1997b) The New Zealand priority criteria project. Part 2: Coronary artery bypass graft surgery, *British Medical Journal*, 314: 135–8.

Ham, C. (1993) priority setting in the NHS: reports from six districts, *British Medical Journal*, 307: 435–8.

Ham, C. (1995) Synthesis: what can we learn from international experience?, in R. Maxwell (ed.) *Rationing Health Care*. Edinburgh: Churchill Livingstone.

Ham, C. (1997) priority setting in health care: learning from international experience, *Health Policy*, 42: 49–66.

Ham, C. (1998) Retracing the Oregon trail: the experience of rationing and the Oregon Health Plan, *British Medical Journal*, 316: 1965–9.

Ham, C. (1999) Tragic choices in health care: lessons from the Child B case, *British Medical Journal*, 319: 1258–61.

Ham, C. and Coulter, A. (2000) Where are we now?, in A. Coulter and C. Ham (eds) *The Global Challenge of Health Care Rationing*. Buckingham: Open University Press.

Ham, C. and Coulter, A. (2001) Explicit and implicit rationing: taking responsibility and avoiding blame for health care choices, *Journal of Health Services Research and Policy*, 6(3): 163–9.

Ham, C. and Locock, L. (1998) *International Approaches to priority setting in Health Care: An Annotated Listing of Official and Semi-official Publications. With a Selection of Key Academic References*. Birmingham: Health Services Management Centre, University of Birmingham.

Ham, C. and McIver, S. (2000) *Contested Decisions: priority setting in the NHS*. London: King's Fund.

Ham, C. and Pickard, S. (1998) *Tragic Choices in Health Care: The Story of Child B*. London: King's Fund.

Harriman, D., McArthur, W. and Zelder, M. (1999) *The availability of medical technology in Canada: an international comparative study*, Public Policy Source Paper no. 28. Vancouver, BC: Fraser Institute.

Harrison, S. and Dowswell, G. (2000) The selective use by NHS management of NICE-promulgated guidelines: a new and effective tool for systematic rationing of new therapies?, in A. Miles, J.R. Hampton and B. Hurwitz (eds) *NICE, CHI and the NHS Reforms. Enabling Excellence or Imposing Control?* London: Aesculapius Medical Press.

Harrison, S. and Hunter, D.J. (1994) *Rationing Health Care*. London: Institute for Public Policy Research.

Haycox, A., Bagust, A. and Walley, T. (1999) Clinical guidelines – the hidden cost, *British Medical Journal*, 318: 391–3.

Health Council of the Netherlands (1991) *Medisch handelen op een tweesprong*. The Hague: Health Council of the Netherlands.

Health Council of the Netherlands (2000) *Van implementeren naar leren: het belang van tweerichtingsverkeer tussen praktijk en wetenschap in de gezondheidszorg*. The Hague: Health Council of the Netherlands.

Health Funding Authority (1998) *How Shall We Prioritize Health and Disability Services?* Wellington: Health Funding Authority.

Health Funding Authority (1999a) HFA interim decisions on the allocation of the 2000/01 sustainable funding path budget increase: Summary of demand driven and new initiative proposals. Unpublished internal report, Health Funding Authority, Wellington, 24 December.

Health Funding Authority (1999b) Report to the Ministry of Health on two Prioritization Demonstration Projects. Unpublished internal report, Health Funding Authority, Wellington, December.

Health Funds Association of New Zealand (1999) *An Insight into the New Zealand Health Insurance Industry*. Wellington: HFANZ Inc.

Health Mo (1997) *Om lov om endringer i folketrygdloven og i enkelte andre lover (bidrag til behandling i utlandet og fylkeskommunens plikt til dekning av behandlingsutgifter)*. Oslo: Ministry of Health.

Heclo, H. (1974) *Modern Social Politics in Britain and Sweden.* New Haven, CT: Yale University Press.

Hefford, B. and Holmes, A. (1999) Booking systems for elective services: the New Zealand experience (with discussion), *Australian Health Review*, 22(4): 61–77.

Heginbotham, C. (1992) Rationing, in R. Smith (ed.) *The Future of Health Care.* London: BMJ Publishing.

Helsedirektoratet (1992) *Benmargstransplantasjon i Norge.* Helsedirektoratets utredningsserie 6–92. Olso: Helsedirektoratet.

Hemminki, E., Hailey, D. and Koivusalo, M. (1999) The courts – a challenge to health technology assessment, *Science Magazine*, 285(5425): 203–4.

Hernes, G. (1996) *Brystkreftsaken og de menneskelige sider.* Aftenposten, 17 July.

Holm, S. (1998) The second phase of priority setting. Goodbye to the simple solutions: the second phase of priority setting in health care, *British Medical Journal*, 317(7164): 1000–2.

Holm, S. (2000) Developments in the Nordic countries – goodbye to the simple solutions, in A. Coulter and C. Ham (eds) *The Global Challenge of Health Care Rationing.* Buckingham: Open University Press.

Holmen, J. (1993) *Høyt blodtrykk. NSAM's handlingsprogram.* Oslo: Folkehelsa.

Holte, H., Kvaløy, S.O., Engan, T., *et al.* (1996) Høydosebehandling med autolog stamcellestøtte ved maligne lidelser, *Tidsskrift for den Norske Lægeforening*, 116(21): 2577–81.

Honigsbaum, F., Calltorp, J., Ham, C. and Holmström, S. (1995) *priority setting Processes for Healthcare.* Oxford: Radcliffe Medical Press.

Honigsbaum, F., Holmström, S. and Calltrop, J. (1997) *Making Choices for Health Care.* Oxford: Radcliffe Medical Press.

Hope, T., Hicks, N., Reynolds, D.J.M., Crisp, R. and Griffiths, S. (1998) Rationing and the health authority, *British Medical Journal*, 317: 1067–9.

House of Commons Select Committee on Health (1999) *Minutes of Evidence for Thursday 4 February 1999. National Institute for Clinical Excellence: Professor Sir Michael Rawlins; Dr Gina Radford and Dr Timothy Riley*, HC 222-i, session 1998–99. London: The Stationery Office. www.parliament.the-stationery-office.co.uk/pa/cm199899/cmselect/cmhealth/222/9020401.htm (accessed 22 August 2002).

House of Commons Select Committee on Health (2002) National Institute for Clinical Excellence. Second report of Session, 2001–02. Volume I: Report and Proceedings of the Committee, HC 515–I, London: The Stationery Office.

Howe, D.T., Gornall, R., Wellesley, D., Boyle, T. and Barber, J. (2000) Six year survey of screening for Down's syndrome by maternal age and mid-trimester ultrasound scans, *British Medical Journal*, 320: 606–10.

Howell, J.B.L. (1992) Re-examining the fundamental principles of the NHS, in R. Smith (ed.) *The Future of Health Care*, London: BMJ Publishing.

Høybråten, D. (2000) Prioriteringer ved et tidsskille. *Dagbladet*, 3 January.

Hunter, D.J. (1993) *Rationing Dilemmas in Health Care.* Birmingham: National Association of Health Authorities and Trusts.

Hunter, D.J. (1995) Rationing health care: the political perspective, *British Medical Journal*, 51: 876–84.

Hunter, D.J. (1997). *Desperately Seeking Solutions. Rationing Health Care.* Harlow: Addison Wesley Longman.

Jacobs, L., Marmor, T. and Oberlander, J. (1999) The Oregon Health Plan and the political paradox of rationing: what advocates and critics have claimed and what Oregon did, *Journal of Health Politics, Policy and Law*, 24(1): 161–80.

Jones, L. (1993) *The Core Debator.* Wellington: National Advisory Committee on Core Health and Disability Support Services.

Jonsen, A.R. and Toulmin, S. (1988) *The Abuse of Casuistry: A History of Moral Reasoning.* Berkeley: University of California Press.

Karlsen, K. (1993) Oslo-lege (53) for gammel for behandling: Dømt til døden av helsevesenet. *Dagbladet*, 5 March.

Kelly, C.A., Harvey, R.J. and Cayton, H. (1997) Drug treatments for Alzheimer's disease [editorial], *British Medical Journal*, 314(7082): 693–4.

Klazinga, N.S. (1994). Compliance with practice guidelines: clinical autonomy revisited, *Health Policy*, 28: 51–66.

Klazinga, N.S. (2000) *Sociale geneeskunde: de derde weg.* Amsterdam: Vossiuspers AUP. www.aup.nl/pdf/ *or* Klazinga.pdf

Klein, R. (1992). Dilemmas and decisions, *Health Management Quarterly*, XIV: 2–5.

Klein, R. (1998). Puzzling about priorities. Why we must acknowledge that rationing is a political process, *British Medical Journal*, 317: 959–60.

Klein, R. and Williams, A. (2000) Setting priorities: what is holding us back – inadequate information or inadequate institutions?, in A. Coulter and C. Ham (eds) *The Global Challenge of Health Care Rationing.* Buckingham: Open University Press.

Klein, R., Day, P. and Redmayne, S. (eds) (1996) *Managing Scarcity.* Buckingham: Open University Press.

Kmietowicz, Z. (2001) Reform of NICE needed to boost its credibility, *British Medical Journal*, 323: 1324.

Kolstad, A., Holte, H., Kvaløy, S. *et al.* (1996) Høydosebehandling med autolog stamcellesøtte ved malignt lymfom og cancer mammae. Erfaring med hematopoetiske stamceller høstet fra blod, *Tidsskrift for den Norske Lægeforening*, 116(21): 2547–51.

Kosecoff, J., Kanouse, D.E., Rogers, W.H. *et al.* (1987) Effects of the National Institutes of Health consensus development program on physician practice, *Journal of the American Medical Association*, 258: 2708–13.

Kreftforening IffoDN (1999) *Cytostatika. Medikamentell kreftbehandling, 5th edition.* Oslo.

Kristoffersen, M. and Piene, H. (1997a) Ventelistegarantiordningen:

Variasjon i andel som får ventelistegaranti, *Tidsskrift for den Norske Lægeforening*, 117(3): 361–5.

Kristoffersen, M. and Piene, H. (1997b) Kriterier for å få ventelistegaranti. Forsøk på presisering, *Tidsskrift for den Norske Lægeforening*, 117(3): 358–61.

Latour, B. (1997) Socrates' and Callicles' settlement or, The invention of the impossible body politic, *Configurations*, 5: 189–240.

Laurance, J. (2000) Alzheimer drugs 'too expensive for NHS', *The Independent*, 12 October.

Lenaghan, J. (1999) The economics of the NHS: assessing the cases for explicit or implicit rationing. Paper presented to the 'priority setting in the NHS' conference, London, 21 September.

Lian, O.S. and Kristiansen, I.S. (1998) Ventetidsgarantien mellom medisin og byråkrati, *Tidsskrift for den Norske Lægeforening*, 118(25): 3921–6.

Lie, R. (1994) Experimental treatment, values, and rationing, *Social Science and Medicine*, 39: 1011–14.

Little, R. (2002) NHS to fund treatment for 10000 patients with MS, *British Medical Journal*, 324: 316.

Locock, L. (2000) The changing nature of rationing in the UK NHS, *Public Administration*, 78(1): 91–109.

Loughlin, M. (2000) 'Quality' and 'excellence': meaning versus rhetoric, in A. Miles, J.R. Hampton and B. Hurwitz (eds) *NICE, CHI and the NHS Reforms. Enabling Excellence or Imposing Control?* London: Aesculapius Medical Press.

Mansoor, O. and Reid, S. (1999) The future of the immunisation schedule: recommendations of a workshop, *New Zealand Medical Journal*, 112: 52–5.

Martin, D.K. and Singer, P.A. (2000) priority setting and health technology assessment: Beyond evidence-based medicine and cost-effectiveness analysis, in A. Coulter and C. Ham (eds) *The Global Challenge of Health Care Rationing*. Buckingham: Open University Press.

Martin, D.K., Pater, J.L. and Singer, P.A. (2001) Priority setting decisions for new cancer drugs: what rationales are used? *Lancet*, 358: 1676–81.

Martin, D.K., Giacomini, M. and Singer, P.A. (2002) Fairness, accountability for reasonableness, and the views of priority setting decision makers, *Health Policy*, 61(3): 279–90.

Matheson, I. (1996) Høydosebehandling med cytostatika som primær behandling ved brystkreft med spredning, *Tidsskrift for den Norske Lægeforening*, 116(16): 1904–6.

Mayor, S. (2001) Health department to fund interferon beta despite institute's ruling, *British Medical Journal*, 323: 1087.

McDonald, G. (2001) Opening up the NICE debate, *British Medical Journal*, 3 October (http://bmj.com/cgi/eletters/323/7315/743).

McGlynn, E.A., Kosecoff, J. and Brook, R.H. (1990) Format and conduct of consensus development conferences. Multi-nation comparison, *International Journal of Technology Assessment in Health Care*, 6(3): 450–69.

McIver, S. and Ham, C. (2000) Five cases, four actors and a moral: lessons from studies of contested treatment decisions, *Health Expectations*, 3: 114–24.

McIver, S., Baines, D., Ham, C. and McLeod, H. (2000) *Setting priorities and managing demand in the NHS. Lessons for primary care groups and trusts and their equivalent organizations in Scotland and Wales.* Birmingham: Health Services Management Centre, University of Birmingham.

McNee, W. (1999) PHARMAC – making tough decisions, in *PHARMAC. Annual Review for the Year Ended June 1999*. Wellington: PHARMAC.

Mechanic, D. (1995). Dilemmas in rationing health care services: the case for implicit rationing, *British Medical Journal*, 310: 1655–9.

Mechanic, D. (1997) Muddling through elegantly, *Health Affairs*, September/October: 83–92.

Meland, E., Ellekjær, H., Gjelsvik, B. *et al.* (2000) Medikamentell forebyggende av hjerte- og karsykdommer i allmennpraksis, *Tidsskrift for den Norske Lægeforening*, 120: 2643–7.

Melzer, D. (1998) New drug treatment for Alzheimer's disease: lessons for healthcare policy, *British Medical Journal*, 316(7133): 762–4.

Members of the Breast Screening Policy Advisory Group (1998) Population-based breast cancer screening: policy advice for a New Zealand screening programme, *New Zealand Medical Journal*, 111: 138–42.

Minister of Health (1999) *Hansard*, 15 June, vol. 333, cols 224, 226.

Minister of Health (2000) *The New Zealand Health Strategy*. Wellington: Ministry of Health.

Ministry of Health (1997) *Forskrift om ventetidsgaranti*. Oslo: Sosial- og Helsedepartementet.

Ministry of Health (2002) *Health Expenditure Trends in New Zealand, 1980–2000*. Wellington: Ministry of Health.

Morone, J.A. (1992) The bias of American politics: rationing health care in a weak state, *University of Pennsylvania Law Review*, 140(5): 1923–38.

Mulder, J.H. (1997) Terug naar de zorg. Dunning gekanteld, *Medisch Contact*, 39: 1219–20.

Mulder, J.H. (2000) Healthcare rationing in the Netherlands: the need for specific guidelines, *Medical Journal Australia*, 172: 329–31.

Mulligan, J. (1998) Health authority purchasing, in J. Le Grand, N. Mays and J.A. Mulligan (eds) *Learning from the NHS Internal Market. A Review of the Evidence*. London: King's Fund.

National Advisory Committee on Core Health and Disability Support Services (1994) *Core Services 1993/94*. Wellington: NACCHDSS.

National Forum on Health (1997) *Final Report – Volume I. Canadian Health Action: Building the Legacy*. Ottawa: National Forum on Health. www.nfh.hc-sc.gc.ca/publicat/finvol1/1trans.htm

National Health Committee (1996) *Annual Report*. Wellington: National Health Committee.

National Health Committee (1997) *Best of Health 3*. Wellington: National Health Committee.

National Health Committee (1998) *Screening for Colorectal Cancer in New Zealand*. Wellington: National Health Committee.

Naylor, C.D., Baigrie, R.S., Goldman, B.S. and Basinski, A. (1990) Assessment of priority for coronary revascularisation procedures. Revascularisation Panel and Consensus Methods Group, *Lancet*, 336(8710): 310–11.

Naylor, C.D., Levinton, C.M., Wheeler, S. and Hunter, L. (1993) Queuing for coronary surgery during severe supply–demand mismatch in a Canadian referral centre: a case study of implicit rationing, *Social Science and Medicine*, 37: 61–7.

Naylor, C.D., Sykora, K., Jaglal, S.B. and Jefferson, S. (1995) Waiting for coronary artery bypass surgery: population-based study of 8517 consecutive patients in Ontario, Canada. The Steering Committee of the Adult Cardiac Care Network of Ontario, *Lancet*, 346(8990): 1605–9.

Newdick, C. (2001) Strong words, *Health Service Journal*, 5 April: 26–7.

NHS Executive (1999a) *'Faster Access to Modern Treatment': How NICE Appraisal Will Work. A Discussion Paper*. Leeds: NHS Executive.

NHS Executive (1999b) *National Institute for Clinical Excellence: Initial Work Programme*. Health Service Circular HSC 1999/176, 6 August. http://tap.ccta.gov.uk/doh/coin4.nsf

NICE (1999a) Board meeting, 21 July 1999. Appendix G 'Appraisal of Health Technologies'. http//www.nice.org.uk/Embcat.asp?page=oldsite/board/2107/app-g.htm (accessed 8 October 2002).

NICE (1999b) Press release, 1999/006, 27 September.

NICE (1999c) Press release, 6 August.

NICE (1999d) *A Guide to Our Work*. London: NICE

NICE (2000a) *Corporate Plan 2000–2003*. London: NICE.

NICE (2000b) Press release, 2000/004, 31 March.

NICE (2000c) *Guidance on the Use of Liquid Based Cytology for Cervical Screening. Technology Appraisal Guidance – no. 5*. London: NICE.

NICE (2001a) *Guide to the Technology Appraisal Process*. London: NICE.

NICE (2001b) *Guidance for Appellants*. London: NICE.

NICE (2001c) *NICE Appraisal of Beta Interferon and Glatiramer for Multiple Sclerosis. Process to January 2002*. http://www.nice.org.uk

Niessen, L.W., Grijseels, E.W.M. and Rutten, F.F.H. (2000) The evidence-based approach in health policy and health care delivery, *Social Science and Medicine*, 51: 859–69.

Nord, E., Richardson, J., Street, A., Kuhse, H. and Singer, P. (1995) Maximizing health benefits vs. egalitarianism: an Australian survey of health issues, *Social Science and Medicine*, 41: 1429–37.

Nord, E., Pinto, J.L., Richardson, J., Menzel, P. and Ubel, P. (1999) Incorporating societal concerns for fairness in numerical valuations of health programmes, *Health Economics*, 8(1): 25–39.

Norges Offentlige Utredninger (1987) *Retningslinjer for prioritering innen norsk helsetjeneste*, NOU 1987:23. Oslo: Universitetsforlaget.

Norges Offentlige Utredninger (1997a) *Prioritering på ny. Gjennomgang av retningslinjer for prioriteringer innen norsk helsetjeneste*, NOU 1997:18. Oslo: Statens Forvaltningstjeneste.

Norges Offentlige Utredninger (1997b) *Piller, prioritering og politikk*, NOU 1997:7. Oslo: Statens Forvaltningstjeneste.

Norges Offentlige Utredninger (1997c) *Omsorg og kunnskap! Norsk kreftplan*, NOU 1997:20. Oslo: Statens Forvaltningstjeneste.

Norheim, O. (1995) The Norwegian welfare state in transition: rationing and plurality of values as ethical challenges for the health care system, *Journal of Medical Philosophy*, 20(6): 639–55.

Norheim, O. (1996) Limiting access to health care: a contractualist approach to fair rationing. Doctoral dissertation, University of Oslo.

Norheim, O. (1999) Healthcare rationing – are additional criteria needed for assessing evidence based clinical practice guidelines? *British Medical Journal*, 319(7222): 1426–9.

Norheim, O. (2000) Increasing demand for accountability: is there a professional response?, in A. Coulter and C. Ham (eds) *The Global Challenge of Health Care Rationing*. Buckingham: Open University Press.

Norheim, O., Ekeberg, O., Evensen, S.A., Halvorsen, M. and Kvernebo, K. (1998) How shall we set priorities among experimental treatment methods? *Nord Med*, 113(1): 17–18, 23–4.

Norheim, O.F., Fougner, J., Søreide, O., Storm-Mathisen, I. and Strengehagen, E. (2002) Klagenemnda for bidrag til behandling i utlandet, *Tidsskrift for den Norske Lægeforening*, 122(16): 1560–3.

Norwegian Consensus Conference on Mammography (1991) Consensus statement, *International Journal of Technology Assessment in Health Care*, 7(1): 84–90.

Norwegian Medicines Agency (1999) *Norwegian Guidelines for Pharmacoeconomic Analysis in connection with Application for Reimbursement*. Oslo: Norwegian Medicines Agency, Department of Pharmacoeconomics.

Nylenna, M. (1995) Norway's decentralized, single-payer health system faces great challenges, *Journal of the American Medical Association*, 274(2): 120–4.

Nylenna, M., Haug, C. and Bjørndal, A. (1996) Høydosebehandling med stamcellestøtte og statsrådstøtte, *Tidsskrift for den Norske Lægeforening*, 116(21): 2537–9.

Oortwijn, W.J. (2000). *First Things First. Priority Setting for Health Technology Assessment*. Amsterdam: Dept. of Epidemiology and Biostatistics/ Institute for Research in Extramural Medicine, Vrije Universiteit Amsterdam.

Oortwijn, W.J. and Mulder, J.H. (2000) *Proceedings of the Third International Conference on Priorities in Health Care*, 22–24 November, Amsterdam. Leiden: Royal Dutch Medical Association.

PaussJensen, A.M., Singer, P.A. and Detsky, A.S. (2002) How Ontario's Formulary Committee makes recommendations. *Pharmacoeconomics*.

Peet, J. (2002) A survey of the Netherlands, *The Economist*, 4 May: 1–18.

Petersen, H., Hilt, B. and Kaasa, S. (1999) Sykefravær mens man står på venteliste, *Tidsskrift for den Norske Lægeforening*, 119(21): 3137–9.

PHARMAC (1999a) *Annual Review for the Year Ended June 1999.* Wellington: PHARMAC.

PHARMAC (1999b) *A Prescription for Pharmacoeconomic Analysis, Version 1.* Wellington: PHARMAC. www.pharmac.govt.nz/pubs/index.html

PHARMAC (2001) *Annual Review for the Year Ended June 2001.* Wellington: PHARMAC.

Piene, H. (1998) Ventetids og behandlingsgarantier – en mur av uvilje? *Tidsskrift for den Norske Lægeforening*, 118(25): 3920.

Piene, H., Hauge, H.K. and Nyen, P.A. (1997) Ventelistegaranti og køer i helsevesenet: Noen teoretiske refleksjoner, *Tidsskrift for den Norske Lægeforening*, 117(3): 370–4.

Pierson, P. (1994) *Dismantling the Welfare State.* Cambridge: Cambridge University Press.

Raftery, J. (2001) NICE: faster access to modern treatments? Analysis of guidance on health technologies, *British Medical Journal*, 323: 1300–3.

Rao, J. (1998) Politicians, not doctors, must make decisions about rationing, *British Medical Journal*, 318: 940.

Rasmussen, K., Haga, D., Larsen, M.L. *et al.* (1997) Et alternativ til dagens ventelistegarantisystem, *Tidsskrift for den Norske Lægeforening*,117(15): 2210–3.

Rawlins, M. (1999a) In pursuit of quality: the National Institute for Clinical Excellence, *Lancet*, 353: 1079–82.

Rawlins, M. (1999b) St Paul International Health Care Annual Lecture, 7 September. http://www.nice.org.uk/article.asp?a=336 (accessed 22 August 2002).

Robert, G. and McIver, S. (2001) How health authorities make decisions about priorities for heart disease. Unpublished report, Health Services Management Centre, University of Birmingham.

Robinson, R. (1999) Limits to rationality: economics, economists and priority setting, *Health Policy,* 49(1–2): 13–26.

Rodwin, M.A. (2000) *Promoting Accountable Managed Health Care: The Potential Role for Consumer Voice.* Bloomington: School of Public and Environmental Affairs, Indiana University. www.consumerfed.org/hmoreport.pdf

Rolstad, K. (1997) Norway, in F. Honigsbaum, S. Holmström and J. Calltorp (eds) *Making Choices for Health Care.* Oxford: Radcliffe Medical Press.

Rosen, R. (1999) Can NICE influence the diffusion of new technologies?, in J. Appleby and A. Harrison (eds) *Health Care UK 1999/2000. The King's Fund Review of Health Policy.* London: King's Fund.

Royal College of Physicians (1995) *Setting Priorities in the NHS. A Framework for Decision-Making.* London: Royal College of Physicians.

Rutten, F. (2000) Interpretatie en gebruik van kosteneffectiviteitsanalyse, in
M. Rutten-van Mölken, J. Busschbach and F. Rutten (eds) *Van Kosten tot
Effecten: Een Handleiding voor Evaluatiesstudies in de Gezondheidszorg*.
Maarssen: Elsevier Gezondheidszorg.

Sabin, J. (1998) Fairness as a problem of love and the heart: a
clinician's perspective on priority setting, *British Medical Journal*,
317:1000–7.

Sculpher, M., Drummond, M. and O'Brien, B. (2001) Effectiveness,
efficiency and NICE, *British Medical Journal*, 322: 943–4.

Singer, P.A. (1997) Resource allocation: beyond evidence-based medicine
and cost-effectiveness analysis, *American College of Physicians Journal
Club*, 127(3): A16–A18.

Singer, P.A., Martin, D.K., Giacomini, M. and Purdy, L. (2000) priority
setting for new technologies in medicine: a qualitative study, *British
Medical Journal*, 321: 1316–18.

Skegg, D., Paul, C., Benson-Cooper, D. *et al.* (1988) Mammographic
screening for breast cancer: prospects for New Zealand. *New Zealand
Medical Journal*, 101: 531–3.

Skogstrøm, L. (1997) Osteoporose-medisiner: Forskere frykter unyttig bruk,
Aftenposten (Morgen), 6 November.

Skouen, J.S., Wester, K. and Slattebrekk, O.V. (1989) What do the waiting
lists cost? A study of patients with backache, *Tidsskrift for den Norske
Lægeforening*, 109(31): 3235–8.

Smith, R. (2000) The failings of NICE, *British Medical Journal*, 321: 1363–4.

SMM (1999a) *The Norwegian Centre for Health Technology Assessment*.
Oslo: Sintef Unimed.

SMM (1999b) *Screening for prostate cancer – An evaluation of available
documentation on medical effects from prostate cancer screening*. Report
No. 3. Oslo: Sintef Unimed.

SMM (1999c) *Thrombolytic medication in the treatment of stroke – A
summary of the state of the art with respect to medical effect of the
treatment*. Report No. 2. Oslo: Sintef Unimed.

SMM (2000) *Heart laser treatment*. Report No. 6. Oslo: Sintef Unimed.

Somdalen, A. (1996) Ingrid Matheson: . . . har du sett hva som står om deg
i avisen i dag? *Tidsskrift for den Norske Lægeforening*, 116: 2594–5.

Søreide, O. and Førde, O.H. (1998) Medisinsk metodevurdering – ny
tvangstrøye eller forsvar for fagligheten? *Tidsskrift for den Norske
Lægeforening*, 118: 4062.

Sosial- og Helsedepartementet (1997) *Forskrift om ventetidsgaranti*. Oslo:
Sosial- og Helsedepartementet.

Sosial- og Helsedepartementet (1998a) *Innsatsstyrt finansiering (ISF) – en
orientering om ordningen og tenkningen rundt ordningen*. Oslo: Sosial- og
Helsedepartementet.   http://odin.dep.no/odinarkiv/norsk/dep/shd/1998/
publ/030005-990107/index-dok000-b-n-a.html   (accessed   10   October
2002).

Sosial- og Helsedepartementet (1998b) *Ot. Prp. nr 12 (1998–99) Lov om pasientrettigheter (pasientrettighetsloven)*. Oslo: Sosial- og Helse-departementet.

Sosial- og Helsedepartementet (1999a) *St. meld. nr. 26 (1999–2000) Om verdiar for den norske helsetenesta*. Oslo: Sosial- og Helsedepartementet.

Sosial- og Helsedepartementet (1999b) *Forskrift om bidrag til behandling i utlandet og om klagenemd for bidrag til behandling i utlandet*. Oslo: Fastsatt av Sosial- og Helsedepartementet.

Statens Helsetilsyn (1994) *Organisering av gastroenterologisk cancerkirurgi i Norge*, Helsetilsynets utredningsserie 6–94. Olso: Statens Helsetilsyn.

Statens Helsetilsyn (1995) *Høydosebehandling med autolog stamcellestøtte ved maligne lidelser*, Helsetilsynets utredningsserie 1–95. Olso: Statens Helsetilsyn. (http://www.helsetilsynet.no/trykksak/ik-2653/innholdsfortegnelse.htm)

Statens Helsetilsyn (1998) *Retningslinjer for retningslinjer. Prosess og metode for utvikling og implementering av faglige retningslinjer*. Oslo: Statens Helsetilsyn.

Stavrum, K. (1997) Pille-firma vil nekte staten ytringsfrihet, *Aftenposten*, 13 November.

Stavrum, K. (1998) Tilbyr medisin mot Alzheimer, *Aftenposten,* 3 April.

Stevens, A., Colin-Jones, D. and Gabbay, J. (1995) 'Quick and clean': authoritative health technology assessment for local health care contracting, *Health Trends*, 27(2): 37–42.

Stolk, E.A., Brouwer, W.B.F. and Busschbach, J.J.V. (2000a) Vergoeding van Viagra stuit op waarden en normen, *Medisch Contact*, 55: 626–9.

Stolk, E.A., Busschbach, J.J.V., Caffa, M., Meuleman, E.J.H. and Rutten, F.F.H. (2000b) Cost utility analysis of sildenafil compared with papaverine-phentolamine injections, *British Medical Journal,* 320: 1165.

Strosberg, M., Wiener, J., Baker, R. and Fein, I. (eds) (1992) *Rationing America's Medical Care: The Oregon Plan and Beyond*. Washington, DC: The Brookings Institution.

Swedish Parliamentary Priorities Commission (1995) *Priorities in Health Care: Ethics, Economy, Implementation*. Stockholm: Ministry of Health and Social Affairs.

Timmins, N. (2000a) The NICE way to bring life to the NHS, *Financial Times*, 20 November.

Timmins, N. (2000b) Secrecy over drug appraisals may end, *Financial Times*, 24–5 June.

Tymstra, T. and Andela, M. (1993) Opinions of Dutch physicians, nurses, and citizens on health care policy, rationing, and technology, *Journal of the American Medical Association*, 270: 2995–9.

Ubel, P.A. and Loewenstein, G. (1995) The efficacy and equity of retrans-plantation: an experimental survey of public attitudes, *Health Policy*, 34: 145–51.

Ubel, P.A., DeKay, M.L., Baron, J. and Asch, D.A. (1996a) Cost-effectiveness analysis in a setting of budget constraints: is it equitable? *New England Journal of Medicine,* 334: 1174–7.

Ubel, P.A., Loewenstein, G., Scanlon, D. and Kamlet, M. (1996b) Individual utilities are inconsistent with rationing choices: a partial explanation of why Oregon's cost-effectiveness list failed, *Medical Decision Making*, 16: 108–16.

Ugnat, A.M. and Naylor, C.D. (1993) Trends in coronary artery bypass grafting in Ontario from 1981 to 1989, *Canadian Medical Association Journal*, 148: 569–75.

van den Burg, M. and ter Meiden, R.H.J. (1998) *Prioriteiten binnen de gezondheidszorg*. Utrecht: Royal Society of Medicine.

van der Grinten, T.E.D. (1996) Scope for policy: essence, operation and reform of the policy of Dutch health care, in L.J. Gunning-Schepers, G.J. Kronjee and R.A. Spasoff (eds) *Fundamental Questions about the Future of Health Care*. The Hague: SDu Uitgevers.

van der Grinten, T.E.D. (2000) Actors in priority setting: intended roles and actual behaviour. Keynote paper presented to the Third International Conference on Priorities in Health Care, Amsterdam.

van der Grinten, T.E.D. and Kasdorp, J.P. (1999) Choices in Dutch health care: mixing strategies and responsibilities, *Health Policy*, 50: 105–22.

van Hout, B., Goes, E.S., Grijseels, E.W.M. and Quarles van Ufford, M.A. (1999) Economic evaluation in the field of cardiology: theory and practice, *Progress in Cardiovascular Diseases,* 42: 167–73.

van Rossum, W. (1991) Decision-making and medical technology assessment: three Dutch cases, *Knowledge and Policy*, 4: 107–24.

Waldenström, U. (1995) A Norwegian consensus on ultrasound scanning. Do not screen pregnant women but provide them with information, *Läkartidningen*, 92(19): 2017–18.

Weaver, K. (1986) The politics of blame avoidance, *Journal of Public Policy*, 6(4): 371–98.

Weggeman, M. (1997) *Kennis management*. Schiedam: Scriptum Management.

Western Canada Waiting List Project (2001) *From Chaos to Order: Making Sense of Waiting Lists in Canada. Final Report.* Edmonton: WCWL Project, University of Alberta. www.wcwl.org/pages/finalreport.pdf

Woolf, S., Grol, R., Hutchinson, A., Eccles, M. and Grimshaw, J. (1999) Potential benefits, limitations and harms of clinical guidelines, *British Medical Journal*, 318: 527–30.

Worth, C. (1999) Use of representative health panel shows changes in public attitudes to rationing, *British Medical Journal*, 318: 940.

Yamey, G. (1999) Chairman of NICE admits that its judgements are hard to defend, *British Medical Journal*, 319: 1222.

Zweibel, N.R., Cassel, C.K. and Karrison, T. (1993) Public attitudes about the use of chronological age as a criterion for allocating health care resources, *The Gerontologist,* 33: 74–80.

INDEX

HEALTH CARE REFORM
LEARNING FROM INTERNATIONAL EXPERIENCE

Chris Ham (ed.)

If you want a broad introduction to international health care reform, written by some of the best health policy analysts alive today, then this is it.

Chris Heginbotham

- What policies have been adopted to reform health care in Europe and North America?
- Which policies have worked and which have failed?
- What new initiatives are emerging onto the health policy agenda?

This book provides an up-to-date review and analysis of health care reform in five countries: Germany, Sweden, the Netherlands, the United Kingdom and the United States. It reviews the experience of introducing competition into the health service as well as policies to strengthen management and change methods of paying hospitals and doctors. The experience of each country is described by experts from the countries concerned. In this lucid introduction, Chris Ham sets out the context of reform, and in the conclusion identifies the emerging lessons.

The book provides an authoritative introduction to health care reform in Europe and North America at a time of increasing political and public interest in this field. It has been designed for students of social policy and the full range of health service practitioners on courses of professional training.

Contents
The background – The United States – The United Kingdom – Sweden – The Netherlands – Germany – Lessons and conclusions – Index.

Contributors
Reinhard Busse, Chris Ham, Bradford Kirkman-Liff, Clas Rehnberg, Freidrich Wilhelm Scwartz and Wynand van de Ven.

160pp   0 335 19889 9 (Paperback)   0 335 19890 2 (Hardback)

THE GLOBAL CHALLENGE OF HEALTH CARE RATIONING

Angela Coulter and Chris Ham (eds)

Rationing or priority setting occurs in all health care systems. Doctors, managers and politicians are involved in making decisions on how to use scarce resources and which groups and patients should receive priority. These decisions may be informed by the results of medical research and cost-effectiveness studies but they also involve the use of judgement and experience. Consequently, priority setting involves ethics as well as economics and decisions on who should live and who should die remain controversial and contested.

This book seeks to illuminate the debate on priority setting by drawing on experience from around the world. The authors are all involved in priority setting, either as decision makers or researchers, and their contributions demonstrate in practical terms how different countries and disciplines are approaching the allocation of resources between competing claims. Accessible to general readers a well as specialists, *The Global Challenge of Health Care Rationing* summarizes the latest thinking in this area and provides a unique resource for those searching for a guide through the maze.

Contents
Introduction – Part 1: How to set priorities – Part 2: Governments and rationing – Part 3: Priorities in developing countries – Part 4: Ethical dilemmas – Part 5: Techniques for determining priorities – Part 6: Involving the public – Part 7: Rationing specific treatments – Conclusion – References – Index.

c. 228 pp   0 335 20463 5 (Paperback)   0 335 20464 3 (Hardback)

USING HEALTH ECONOMICS IN HEALTH SERVICES
RATIONING RATIONALITY?

Ruth McDonald

Using Health Economics in Health Services examines the impact of attempts to use 'rational' health economic analyses on local decision making in the National Health Service. The book presents findings from an ethnographic study of one Health Authority and one Primary Care Group to present a rich picture of the processes and contexts of health care resource allocation at local level.

The conclusion of the book is that it is extremely difficult to use 'rational' solutions to resource allocation dilemmas at local level in the modern state. The adoption by local decision makers of what appear to be non-rational coping strategies is essential to the maintenance of service delivery in the context of resource scarcity. Paradoxically, attempts to impose 'rational' decision making threaten to undermine the precarious stability of the very systems they seek to improve. In this sense, the pursuit of rationality may itself be an irrational act.

Written in an engaging and lively style, the book will be accessible to general readers as well as specialists in the field. It has been designed for use by students of health economics, health policy, public administration and health services management and will be of interest to practitioners and researchers in these fields.

Contents
Series editor's preface – List of tables – List of abbreviations – Introduction and methods – Rational decision making and health economics – The Health Authority context: an overview – Case study I: a cost effectiveness analysis of cholesterol lowering drugs – Case study II: system wide modelling of CHD services in Poppleton Health Authority – Case study III: statins, heart failure and chest pain in Baxby – Towards understanding – Bibliography – Index.

208pp   0 335 20983 1 (Paperback)   0 335 20984 X (Hardback)

MANAGING SCARCITY
PRIORITY SETTING AND RATIONING IN THE NATIONAL HEALTH SERVICE

Rudolf Klein, Patricia Day and Sharon Redmayne

The 'rationing' of health care has become one of the most emotive issues of the 1990s in the UK, causing much public confusion and political controversy. This book provides a comprehensive and critical introduction to this debate. It does so by examining the processes which determine who gets what in the way of treatment, the decision makers involved at different levels in the NHS and the criteria used in making such decisions. In particular it analyses the relationship between decisions about spending priorities (taken by politicians and managers) and decisions about rationing care for individual patients (taken by doctors), between explicit and implicit rationing. As well as drawing on research-based evidence about what is happening in Britain today, *Managing Scarcity* also looks at the experience of the NHS since 1948 and puts the case of health care in the wider context of publicly funded services and programmes which have to allocate limited resources according to non-market criteria.

Managing Scarcity is recommended reading for students and researchers of health policy, as well as health professionals and policy makers at all levels in the NHS.

Contents
Part 1: The context – Unpicking the notion – Politics and strategies – Principles of resource allocation – Part 2: The NHS experience – The NHS: a history of institutionalized scarcity – Priority setting in the new era – Lifting the veils from rationing? – Into the secret garden – Part 3: The way ahead – Money or science to the rescue? – What can we learn from the others? – Policy options for the future – Appendix – References – Index.

176pp   0 335 19446 X (Paperback)   0 335 19447 8 (Hardback)